HEALTHY VEGETABLE RECIPES FOR BEGINNERS

Your Essential Guide to Seasonal, Local, and Sustainable Cooking

By

Hector Wiggins

Table of Contents

INTRODUCTION

Greetings from the realm of nutritious food! Making the decision to increase your intake of vegetables is a great first step toward improved health and wellness. This booklet, "Healthy Vegetable Recipes for Beginners," is intended to help you navigate the fascinating world of plant-based food, regardless of your level of experience in the kitchen.

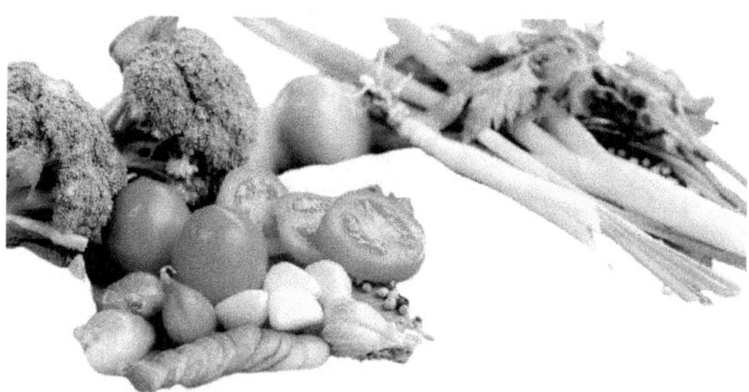

In the hectic world of today, it can be simple to underestimate the value of eating a wide range of vegetables. However, these nutrient-dense powerhouses are necessary to keep your body at its best. Vegetables are a great source of vitamins, minerals, fiber, and antioxidants. They can also help with weight management, digestion, and lower the risk of chronic illnesses like diabetes, heart disease, and some types of cancer. Adopting a diet heavy in vegetables not only nourishes your health but also promotes animal welfare and environmental sustainability.

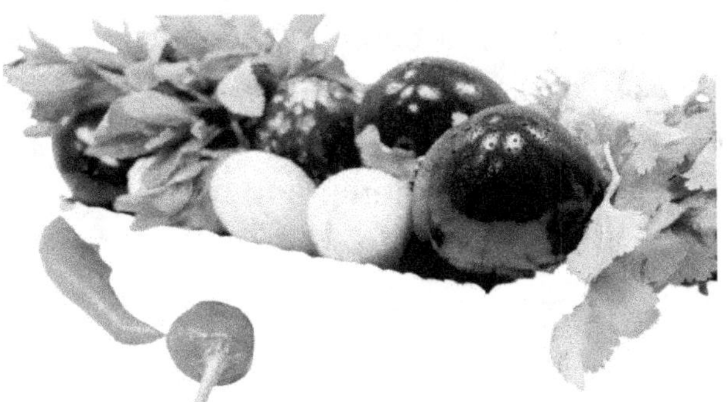

This handbook offers a gentle introduction to the world of vegetable-based cuisine and is designed exclusively for novices. You'll find a ton of delectable and approachable recipes to motivate you on your path, whether you're switching to a vegetarian or vegan lifestyle or just trying to eat more plant-based foods.

Let's take time to become comfortable with a few kitchen necessities before getting started with the recipes. Possessing the appropriate tools and pantry essentials can position you for success in the kitchen, from fundamental utensils and tools to necessary components. If you're new to cooking, don't worry—many of the recipes in this book are ideal for novices as they call for basic ingredients and methods.

The amazing range of flavors, textures, and colors that veggies provide is one of the most fascinating things about cooking with vegetables. A universe of culinary possibilities awaits exploration, ranging from fragrant stir-fries and savory roasts to crisp salads and robust soups.This cookbook has something to suit every palate, whether it's for a hearty bowl of soup on a cold night or a light and refreshing lunch.

Every recipe in this book has been hand-picked , tried and tested to make sure it's not only delicious but also suitable for beginners. You'll be empowered to confidently prepare tasty and nourishing meals by following the step-by-step directions along with useful tips and tricks. Furthermore, you won't have to bother looking for hard-to-find goods because you can find all the components you need at your neighborhood grocery store or farmers' market.

Remember to approach cooking with an open mind and a spirit of inquiry as you set off on this culinary adventure. Try different flavors and ingredients without fear, and don't let the odd failure deter you from trying new things. Following recipes is just as important to cooking as using your imagination and exploring new flavors. Now let's begin cooking, put on your sleeves, and sharpen your knives!

Benefits of Eating Vegetables

The benefits of eating vegetables are wide-ranging and encompass various aspects of physical health, mental well-being, and environmental sustainability. Here's a comprehensive explanation of these benefits:

Nutrient Density: Vegetables are packed with essential nutrients such as vitamins, minerals, fiber, and antioxidants. These nutrients are vital for supporting overall health, immune function, and disease prevention. Consuming a diverse range of vegetables ensures that your body receives a wide spectrum of nutrients necessary for optimal functioning.

Disease Prevention: Numerous studies have shown that diets rich in vegetables are associated with a reduced risk of chronic diseases such as heart disease, stroke, diabetes, and certain types of cancer.

The high levels of antioxidants found in vegetables help protect cells from damage caused by free radicals, thereby reducing inflammation and lowering the risk of developing chronic conditions.

Weight management: Vegetables are a great option for people trying to control their weight because they are high in fiber and low in calories. Vegetables' high fiber content contributes to satiety, making you feel full and content for longer periods of time. This lowers the risk of overeating and supports attempts to lose or maintain weight.

Digestive Health: The fiber found in vegetables plays a crucial role in supporting digestive health by promoting regularity and preventing constipation. Additionally, certain vegetables contain prebiotics, which nourish beneficial gut bacteria and contribute to a healthy gut microbiome.

A healthy gut microbiome is associated with improved digestion, nutrient absorption, and immune function.

Heart Health: Vegetables, particularly leafy greens and cruciferous vegetables like broccoli and Brussels sprouts, are rich in heart-healthy nutrients such as potassium, magnesium, and folate. These nutrients help regulate blood pressure, reduce cholesterol levels, and support overall cardiovascular health, lowering the risk of heart disease and stroke.

Improved Mood and Mental Well-being: Eating a diet rich in vegetables has been linked to improved mood, mental clarity, and cognitive function. The nutrients found in vegetables, such as folate, vitamin B6, and antioxidants, play a role in neurotransmitter synthesis and brain function, potentially reducing the risk of depression and cognitive decline.

Hydration and Detoxification: Many vegetables have high water content, which helps keep the body hydrated and supports proper hydration levels.Additionally, certain vegetables, such as leafy greens and cruciferous vegetables, contain compounds that support the body's natural detoxification processes, helping to eliminate toxins and promote overall detoxification.

Environmental Sustainability: Choosing to incorporate more vegetables into your diet is not only beneficial for your health but also for the planet. Plant-based diets have a lower environmental footprint compared to diets high in animal products, as they require fewer resources such as land, water, and energy to produce. By reducing reliance on animal agriculture, which is a significant contributor to greenhouse gas emissions and deforestation, consuming more vegetables helps mitigate environmental degradation and promote sustainability.

Tips for Beginners

Here are detailed tips for beginners looking to explore healthy vegetable recipes:

Start with Familiar Vegetables: Begin your journey into vegetable-based cooking by choosing vegetables that you are already familiar with and enjoy eating. This can help make the transition to vegetarian meals feel less daunting and more enjoyable. Common options like carrots, spinach, bell peppers, and tomatoes are versatile and easy to incorporate into various dishes.

Experiment with Different Cooking Methods: Explore a variety of cooking methods to discover new flavors and textures. Experiment with roasting, grilling, sautéing, steaming, and even raw preparations to see which methods you prefer. Each cooking technique can bring out unique qualities in vegetables and add depth to your dishes.

Embrace Seasonal Produce: Incorporating seasonal produce into your meals not only ensures freshness and flavor but also supports local farmers and reduces environmental impact. Visit farmers' markets or join a community-supported agriculture (CSA) program to access a diverse selection of seasonal vegetables. Experimenting with seasonal ingredients can also inspire creativity in the kitchen.

Plan and Prep Ahead: To make vegetable-based cooking more convenient, consider planning and prepping your meals in advance. Spend some time each week washing, chopping, and portioning vegetables so they're ready to use when you need them. Having prepped ingredients on hand can streamline the cooking process and make mealtime preparation quicker and easier.

Don't Fear Spices and Herbs: Spices and herbs are essential for adding flavor and depth to vegetable dishes. Don't be afraid to experiment with different combinations of spices and herbs to elevate the taste of your meals. Start with basic options like garlic, onion, black pepper, and parsley, then gradually expand your spice rack as you become more comfortable with flavor pairings.

Balance Flavors and Textures: Aim to create balanced meals that incorporate a variety of flavors and textures. Combine sweet, savory, sour, and spicy elements to create depth of flavor, and incorporate crunchy, creamy, and chewy textures for added interest. Experiment with contrasting flavors and textures to keep your meals exciting and satisfying.

Include Protein and Healthy Fats: To create well-rounded and satisfying vegetable-based meals, ensure that you include sources of protein and healthy fats. Incorporate plant-based protein sources such as beans, lentils, tofu, tempeh, nuts, and seeds into your dishes. Additionally, include healthy fats from sources like avocado, olive oil, nuts, and seeds to provide satiety and support nutrient absorption.

Get Creative with Substitutions: Don't hesitate to get creative with substitutions in recipes to accommodate dietary preferences or ingredient availability. Experiment with swapping out ingredients like pasta for spiralized vegetables, rice for cauliflower rice, or meat for plant-based alternatives. Substitutions can add variety to your meals and open up new culinary possibilities.

Educate Yourself: Take the time to educate yourself about the nutritional benefits of different vegetables and how to properly prepare them. Research cooking techniques, watch tutorial videos, and read cookbooks or online resources to expand your knowledge and skills. The more you learn about vegetables and cooking methods, the more confident you'll become in the kitchen.

Enjoy the Process: Above all, remember to enjoy the process of exploring healthy vegetable recipes. Cooking can be a fun and rewarding experience, so embrace the opportunity to experiment, learn, and create delicious meals that nourish your body and soul. Don't be afraid to make mistakes along the way – they're all part of the learning process. Have fun, be adventurous, and savor the flavors of your culinary creations!

CHAPTER ONE

Kitchen Essentials

Here's a list of kitchen essentials for beginners who are interested in preparing healthy vegetable recipes, along with explanations of their importance:

Chef's Knife: A high-quality chef's knife is essential for chopping, slicing, and dicing vegetables with precision and ease. Look for a knife with a sharp blade and a comfortable handle that feels secure in your hand.

Cutting Board: A sturdy cutting board provides a stable surface for chopping vegetables and prevents damage to your countertops. Opt for a cutting board made of wood or plastic that is easy to clean and maintain.

Vegetable Peeler: A vegetable peeler makes it easy to remove the skins from vegetables like carrots, potatoes, and cucumbers, allowing you to incorporate them into your recipes with ease.

Vegetable Brush: A vegetable brush is useful for scrubbing dirt and debris from the surface of vegetables, especially when using organic produce or vegetables with rough skin like potatoes and carrots.

Mixing Bowls: A set of mixing bowls in various sizes is indispensable for mixing ingredients, tossing salads, and marinating vegetables. Choose bowls made of stainless steel, glass, or ceramic that are durable and easy to clean.

Sauté Pan or Skillet: A sauté pan or skillet is essential for cooking vegetables on the stovetop. Look for a pan with a non-stick surface and a sturdy handle for easy maneuverability.

Sheet Pan: A sturdy sheet pan is perfect for roasting vegetables in the oven. Choose a pan made of heavy-duty aluminum or stainless steel that can withstand high temperatures and won't warp over time.

Blender or Food Processor: A blender or food processor is useful for preparing smoothies, sauces, soups, and dips using a variety of vegetables. Look for a model with multiple speeds and attachments for versatility.

Steamer Basket: A steamer basket allows you to cook vegetables gently by steaming, preserving their nutrients and natural flavors. Opt for a collapsible steamer basket that fits easily into your pots and pans.

Measuring Cups and Spoons: Accurate measuring cups and spoons are essential for following recipes and portioning ingredients properly. Look for a set that includes both dry and liquid measurements for versatility.

Oven Mitts or Pot Holders: Protect your hands from burns and injuries while handling hot pans and baking sheets with oven mitts or pot holders. Choose a pair that is heat-resistant and comfortable to wear.

Kitchen Towels and Dishcloths: Keep your workspace clean and dry with kitchen towels and dishcloths. Use them to wipe up spills, dry washed vegetables, and handle hot pots and pans safely.

By equipping your kitchen with these essential tools, you'll have everything you need to embark on your journey of preparing healthy vegetable recipes with confidence and ease. As you gain experience and explore new recipes, you may find that additional tools and gadgets become useful, but starting with these basics will set you up for success in the kitchen.

Tools and Utensils

Tools and utensils for healthy vegetable recipes typically include:

Chef's Knife: A sharp, high-quality chef's knife is essential for chopping, dicing, and slicing vegetables efficiently.

Cutting Board: Use a sturdy cutting board to protect your countertops and provide a stable surface for chopping vegetables.

Vegetable Peeler: This tool helps peel vegetables like carrots, potatoes, and cucumbers, making them ready for cooking or raw consumption.

Vegetable Brush: A brush is handy for cleaning dirt and debris from vegetables like potatoes and root vegetables.

Steamer Basket: Steaming vegetables retains more nutrients compared to boiling or frying. A steamer basket allows you to steam vegetables easily.

Salad Spinner: Essential for washing and drying leafy greens like lettuce and spinach, ensuring they're clean and crisp for salads and other dishes.

Grater or Mandoline: Useful for shredding or thinly slicing vegetables like carrots, zucchini, and cabbage for salads or stir-fries.

Immersion Blender or Food Processor: Great for blending soups, making smoothies, or creating vegetable purees.

Non-Stick Pan or Wok: Ideal for sautéing vegetables with minimal oil, maintaining their nutrients and natural flavors.

Baking Sheet or Roasting Pan: Perfect for roasting a variety of vegetables like sweet potatoes, Brussels sprouts, and cauliflower, enhancing their natural sweetness and flavor.

Herb Mill or Herb Scissors: These tools make it easy to chop fresh herbs like basil, parsley, and cilantro to enhance the flavor of your vegetable dishes.

Tongs and Spatula: Essential for flipping and stirring vegetables while cooking, ensuring even cooking and preventing sticking.

By having these tools and utensils on hand, you'll be well-equipped to prepare a wide range of healthy and delicious vegetable recipes.

Basic Ingredients

The following is an explanation list of staple ingredients for beginner-friendly, healthful vegetable recipes:

Fresh Vegetables: Select a rainbow of vibrant veggies, including tomatoes, bell peppers, and zucchini, as well as cruciferous (broccoli, cauliflower), root (carrots, sweet potatoes), and leafy greens (kale, spinach). These supply vital nutrients, vitamins, and fiber.

Herbs and Spices: Herbs like basil, parsley, cilantro, and spices such as garlic, ginger, cumin, and paprika add flavor to vegetable dishes without adding extra calories. Experimenting with different herbs and spices can elevate the taste of your recipes.

Healthy Oils: Opt for heart-healthy oils like olive oil, avocado oil, or coconut oil for cooking and dressing vegetables. These oils provide healthy fats and can enhance the flavor of your dishes.

Whole Grains: To add texture, fiber, and extra nutrients to your veggie recipes, try using whole grains like quinoa, brown rice, barley, or whole wheat pasta.

Legumes: Chickpeas, lentils, and beans are great providers of fiber and plant-based protein. You may add them to stir-fries, salads, soups, and stews to increase the filling and nutritional value of your vegetable dishes.

Nuts and Seeds: Add crunch and protein to your vegetable dishes by including nuts and seeds like almonds, walnuts, pumpkin seeds, or sesame seeds. They also provide healthy fats and essential nutrients.

Citrus Fruits: Lemon, lime, and orange juice can be used to add acidity and brightness to vegetable dishes. They can be used in dressings, marinades, or simply squeezed over cooked vegetables for extra flavor.

Vinegar: Balsamic vinegar, apple cider vinegar, or rice vinegar can be used to add tanginess to salads, roasted vegetables, or marinades. They can also help balance the flavors of your dishes.

Low-Sodium Broth or Stock: Using vegetable broth or stock as a base for soups, stews, and sauces adds depth of flavor without excess sodium. Look for low-sodium options to control the salt content of your dishes.

Sweeteners: Natural sweeteners like honey, maple syrup, or agave nectar can be used sparingly to balance the flavors of savory vegetable dishes, particularly when roasting or caramelizing vegetables.

CHAPTER TWO

Salad Creations

Salad ideas are flexible and provide countless opportunities for preparing nutritious vegetable foods. Here's how to make scrumptious, wholesome salads:

Base Greens: To begin, lay out a bed of fresh greens, such as romaine lettuce, spinach, kale, or mixed salad greens. These greens are high in fiber, vitamins, and minerals.

Colorful Vegetables: Add a variety of colorful vegetables for flavor, texture, and nutrients. Some options include cherry tomatoes, cucumbers, bell peppers, carrots, radishes, red onions, shredded cabbage, and sugar snap peas.

Protein: Incorporate protein sources to make your salad more satisfying and balanced. Options include grilled chicken breast, sliced turkey or ham, hard-boiled eggs, tofu, chickpeas, black beans, quinoa, or edamame.

Healthy Fats: Include sources of healthy fats to add richness and flavor to your salad. Consider adding avocado slices, nuts (such as almonds, walnuts, or pecans), seeds (such as pumpkin seeds, sunflower seeds, or sesame seeds), or crumbled feta or goat cheese.

Whole Grains: Add cooked whole grains like quinoa, brown rice, farro, barley, or couscous to bulk up your salad and provide complex carbohydrates and additional fiber.

Fruit: Incorporate fresh or dried fruits for a touch of sweetness and added nutrients. Try adding sliced strawberries, blueberries, apples, pears, grapes, or dried cranberries or apricots.

Herbs and Spices: Fresh herbs like basil, cilantro, mint, or parsley can add freshness and flavor to your salad. Sprinkle it with spices like black pepper, cumin, paprika, or chili flakes for extra depth.

Dressing: Choose a homemade or store-bought dressing that complements the flavors of your salad. Opt for vinaigrettes made with olive oil and vinegar or citrus juice, or try creamy dressings made with Greek yogurt or avocado for a healthier option.

Texture: Add crunchy elements like croutons, toasted nuts or seeds, or crispy chickpeas to provide texture contrast to your salad.

Garnish: Finish your salad with a final flourish by adding a garnish such as fresh herbs, grated Parmesan cheese, or a sprinkle of toasted sesame seeds.

Classic Garden Salad

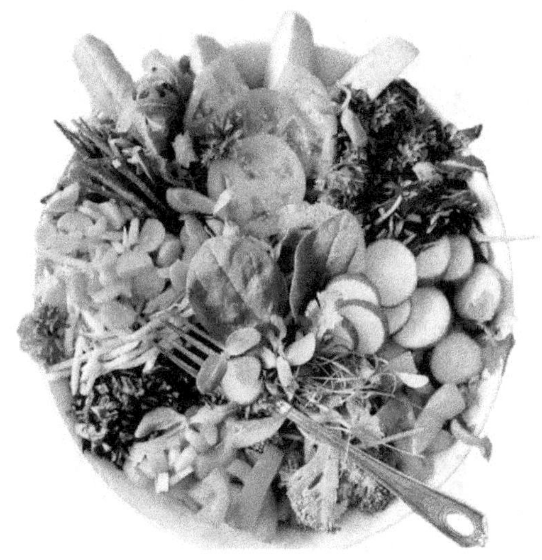

A Classic Garden Salad is a timeless and refreshing dish that showcases a variety of fresh vegetables. Here's how to make one for a healthy vegetable recipe:

Ingredients:
Mixed salad greens (such as lettuce, spinach, arugula)
Cherry tomatoes, halved
Cucumber, sliced
Red onion, thinly sliced
Carrot, shredded or sliced into matchsticks
Bell pepper, thinly sliced
Optional: Radishes, celery, avocado slices.

Dressing:
Olive oil
Balsamic vinegar or red wine vinegar
Dijon mustard
Garlic, minced
Salt and pepper to taste.

Instructions:
Prepare the Vegetables: Wash and dry the salad greens thoroughly. Tear the larger leaves into bite-sized pieces. Slice the cherry tomatoes in half, cucumber into rounds, and thinly slice the red onion and bell pepper. Shred or slice the carrot.

Assemble the Salad: In a large bowl, combine the mixed salad greens with the prepared vegetables. Toss gently to mix evenly.

To prepare the dressing, combine the olive oil, balsamic vinegar, Dijon mustard, minced garlic, salt, and pepper in a small bowl. To suit your own taste, adjust the proportions.

Dress the Salad: Drizzle the dressing over the salad and toss gently to coat the vegetables evenly. Start with a small amount of dressing and add more as needed.

Serve: Transfer the dressed salad to serving plates or a large salad bowl. Optionally, garnish with additional toppings like avocado slices or toasted nuts.

Enjoy: Serve the Classic Garden Salad as a side dish or add protein such as grilled chicken, tofu, or hard-boiled eggs to make it a complete meal. Enjoy the fresh and vibrant flavors of this healthy vegetable recipe!

Feel free to customize the salad by adding or omitting ingredients based on your preferences and what's in season. This Classic Garden Salad is not only delicious but also packed with nutrients, making it a perfect choice for a healthy meal or side dish.

Caesar Salad with Homemade Dressing

A Caesar Salad with Homemade Dressing is a classic dish that can be made healthier by using homemade dressing with wholesome ingredients. Here's how to prepare it:

Ingredients:

For the Salad:
Romaine lettuce, washed and chopped
Grated Parmesan cheese
Whole grain croutons (optional)
Grilled chicken breast, sliced (optional).

For the Dressing:
1/4 cup plain Greek yogurt
2 tablespoons freshly squeezed lemon juice
1 tablespoon Dijon mustard
1 clove garlic, minced
2 anchovy filets (optional, for traditional Caesar flavor)

1/4 cup grated Parmesan cheese
Salt and black pepper to taste
2-3 tablespoons extra virgin olive oil.

Instructions:

Prepare the Salad Ingredients:
Wash and chop the romaine lettuce into
bite-sized pieces.
Grate the Parmesan cheese and prepare the
croutons if using.
Optionally, grill and slice the chicken breast for
added protein.

Make the Dressing:
In a blender or food processor, combine the
Greek yogurt, lemon juice, Dijon mustard,
minced garlic, anchovy filets (if using), grated
Parmesan cheese, salt, and black pepper.
Blend until smooth and well combined.

With the blender or food processor running, slowly drizzle in the olive oil until the dressing reaches the desired consistency. Adjust seasoning to taste.

Assemble the Salad:
In a large salad bowl, toss the chopped romaine lettuce with the grated Parmesan cheese and croutons (if using).
Add the grilled chicken slices if desired.

Dress the Salad:
Drizzle the homemade Caesar dressing over the salad, starting with a small amount and adding more as needed.
Toss the salad gently to evenly coat the lettuce with the dressing.

Serve:
Divide the Caesar Salad into individual serving bowls or plates.
Optionally, garnish with additional grated Parmesan cheese and freshly ground black pepper.

Enjoy:
Serve immediately and enjoy the fresh and flavorful Caesar Salad with Homemade Dressing as a nutritious and satisfying meal or side dish.

By making the dressing from scratch with Greek yogurt and wholesome ingredients, you can create a healthier version of the classic Caesar Salad without sacrificing flavor. Feel free to customize the salad with additional vegetables or protein according to your preferences.

Greek Salad with Feta and Olives

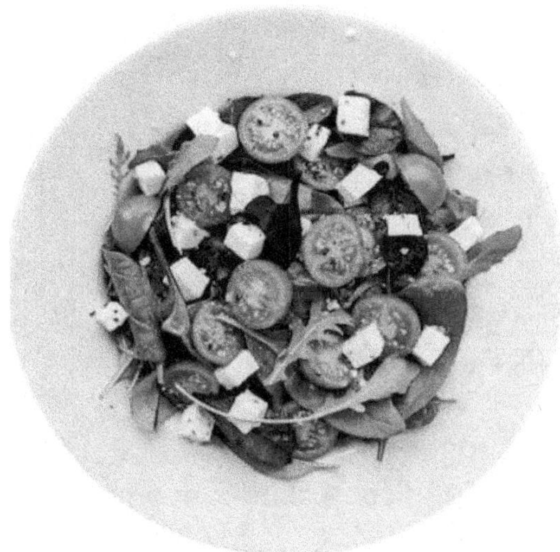

Greek Salad with Feta and Olives is a flavorful and nutritious dish that highlights the fresh flavors of Mediterranean vegetables. Here's how to make it:

Ingredients:
Romaine lettuce or mixed salad greens
Cucumber, sliced
Cherry tomatoes, halved
Red onion, thinly sliced
Kalamata olives, pitted
Feta cheese, crumbled
Optional: Bell pepper, sliced
For the Dressing:
Extra virgin olive oil
Red wine vinegar or lemon juice
Dried oregano
Salt and black pepper to taste
Optional: Minced garlic, for extra flavor.

Instructions:

Get the salad ready. Ingredients: Rinse and pat dry the mixed salad greens or lettuce. Cut the bigger leaves into small pieces using a fork. Cut the bell pepper, if used, into slices, finely slice the red onion, slice the cucumber, and cut the cherry tomatoes in half.

Assemble the Salad:
In a large salad bowl, combine the prepared lettuce or mixed greens with the sliced cucumber, cherry tomatoes, red onion, bell pepper (if using), and Kalamata olives. Crumble the feta cheese over the salad.

Make the Dressing:
In a small bowl, whisk together extra virgin olive oil, red wine vinegar or lemon juice, dried oregano, salt, and black pepper. Adjust the proportions to taste.
Optionally, add minced garlic for extra flavor.

Dress the Salad:
Drizzle the dressing over the salad, starting with a small amount and adding more as needed. Toss the salad gently to coat the vegetables and feta cheese evenly with the dressing.

Serve:
Transfer the Greek Salad with Feta and Olives
to serving plates or a large salad bowl.

Enjoy:
Serve immediately and enjoy the fresh and
vibrant flavors of this healthy vegetable recipe.
Optionally, serve with crusty bread or grilled
chicken for a complete meal.

Greek Salad with Feta and Olives is not only
delicious but also packed with nutrients from
the variety of colorful vegetables and the
healthy fats from the olives and olive oil. It's a
perfect dish for a light and refreshing lunch or
dinner.

Quinoa and Vegetable Salad

Quinoa and Vegetable Salad is a nutritious and versatile dish that combines fluffy quinoa with a variety of fresh vegetables. Here's how to make it:

Ingredients:
Quinoa
Mixed vegetables (such as bell peppers, cucumbers, cherry tomatoes, red onion, carrots, broccoli)
Fresh herbs (such as parsley, cilantro, or basil)
Optional add-ins: avocado, chickpeas, feta cheese, nuts or seeds.

For the Dressing:
Extra virgin olive oil
Lemon juice or vinegar (such as red wine vinegar or apple cider vinegar)
Dijon mustard
Garlic, minced
Salt and pepper to taste.

Instructions:

Cook the Quinoa: To get rid of any bitterness, rinse the quinoa under cool water.
One part quinoa and two parts water or vegetable broth should be combined in a saucepan.
After bringing to a boil, lower the heat to a simmer, cover, and cook the quinoa for 15 to 20 minutes, or until it is tender and the liquid has been absorbed.
Take it off the heat and leave it covered for five minutes. Using a fork, fluff and allow to cool.

Prepare the Vegetables:
Wash and chop the mixed vegetables into bite-sized pieces. You can use any combination of vegetables you like, depending on your preferences and what's in season.
If using broccoli, blanch it in boiling water for 1-2 minutes, then rinse under cold water to stop the cooking process and preserve its vibrant color.

Make the Dressing:
In a small bowl, whisk together the extra virgin olive oil, lemon juice or vinegar, Dijon mustard, minced garlic, salt, and pepper until well combined. Adjust the proportions to taste.

Assemble the Salad:
In a large mixing bowl, combine the cooked quinoa with the chopped vegetables and fresh herbs.
If using optional add-ins like avocado, chickpeas, feta cheese, or nuts/seeds, add them to the bowl as well.

Toss the salad carefully to ensure that all of the components are uniformly coated after adding the dressing. Dressing should be added little at first and more as needed.

Serve:
Transfer the Quinoa and Vegetable Salad to a
serving dish or individual plates.
Optionally, garnish with additional fresh herbs
or a sprinkle of feta cheese or nuts/seeds for
extra flavor and texture.

Enjoy:
Serve the salad immediately as a light and
nutritious meal or side dish. It's perfect for
lunch, dinner, or as a make-ahead option for
meal prep.

A nutritious option for any occasion, quinoa
and vegetable salad is not only tasty and filling
but also high in protein, fiber, vitamins, and
minerals. You are welcome to add your own
vegetables and toppings to the salad to make it
to your own personal choice.

CHAPTER THREE

Soups and Stews

Soups and stews are versatile dishes that can be packed with healthy vegetables, making them an excellent option for nutritious meals. Here's an overview of soups and stews for healthy vegetable recipes:

Benefits of Soups and Stews with Vegetables:

Nutrient-Rich: Soups and stews often contain a variety of vegetables, providing essential vitamins, minerals, and fiber for overall health and well-being.

Hydration: Soups are usually broth-based, which helps keep you hydrated while enjoying a delicious meal, especially important during colder months.

Satiety: The combination of vegetables, protein, and often whole grains or legumes in soups and stews can help keep you feeling full and satisfied for longer periods.

Versatility: You can use a wide range of vegetables in soups and stews, allowing for creativity and variety in your meals. It's a great way to incorporate seasonal produce and use up any vegetables you have on hand.

Meal Prep Friendly: Soups and stews are often even better the next day, making them ideal for meal prep. You can batch cook a large pot and portion it out for easy grab-and-go meals throughout the week.

Tips for Healthy Soups and Stews:
Choose a Variety of Vegetables: Aim to include a colorful array of vegetables in your soups and stews to maximize nutrition and flavor. Consider using carrots, celery, onions, bell peppers, leafy greens, tomatoes, squash, and more.

Use Lean Proteins: Incorporate lean proteins such as chicken breast, turkey, lean beef, fish, tofu, or beans to add satiety and nutritional value to your soups and stews.

Opt for Homemade Broth: Make your own broth or stock using vegetable scraps or leftover bones for added flavor and to control the sodium content. Alternatively, choose low-sodium store-bought options.

Limit Added Fat: While some fat is necessary for flavor and satiety, aim to use healthier fats like olive oil or avocado oil sparingly when sautéing vegetables or browning meats.

Season with Herbs and Spices: Enhance the flavor of your soups and stews with a variety of herbs and spices instead of relying on excess salt. Experiment with combinations like garlic, thyme, rosemary, cumin, paprika, or curry powder.

Bulk Up with Whole Grains or Legumes:
Add cooked whole grains such as quinoa,
brown rice, barley, or farro, or legumes like
lentils, chickpeas, or black beans to increase
the fiber and protein content of your soups and
stews.

**Examples of Healthy Vegetable Soups and
Stews:**
Minestrone Soup with lots of mixed vegetables,
beans, and whole wheat pasta.

Lentil and Vegetable Stew loaded with carrots,
celery, onions, and spinach.

Chicken and Vegetable Soup featuring chicken
breast, carrots, celery, and leafy greens in a
flavorful broth.

Spicy Black Bean and Vegetable Chili with bell
peppers, tomatoes, corn, and spices for a
hearty and satisfying meal.

Healthy Vegetable Soup

A Healthy Vegetable Soup is a nutritious and comforting dish made primarily with vegetables and flavorful broth. Here's how to make one:

Ingredients:
Mixed vegetables (such as carrots, celery, onions, potatoes, tomatoes, bell peppers, zucchini)
Low-sodium vegetable broth or homemade vegetable stock
Garlic, minced
Olive oil or avocado oil
Herbs and spices (such as thyme, rosemary, bay leaves, paprika, black pepper)
Optional: Leafy greens (such as spinach, kale), legumes (such as lentils, beans), whole grains (such as quinoa, barley), protein (such as chicken, tofu).

Instructions:

Prepare the Vegetables:
Wash, peel, and chop the vegetables into
bite-sized pieces. You can use a variety of
vegetables based on your preferences and
what's in season.

Sauté the Aromatics:
In a large soup pot or Dutch oven, heat olive oil
or avocado oil over medium heat.
Add minced garlic and sauté for 1-2 minutes
until fragrant, being careful not to burn it.

Add the Vegetables:
Add the chopped vegetables to the pot, starting
with the ones that take longer to cook (such as
carrots and potatoes) and gradually adding the
rest.
Sauté the vegetables for a few minutes until
they start to soften slightly.

Simmer with Broth: Add just enough homemade vegetable stock or low-sodium vegetable broth to cover the vegetables. If necessary, you can also add water.

To flavor the soup, add any herbs and spices you're using, like black pepper, paprika, bay leaves, thyme, and rosemary.

After bringing the soup to a boil, lower the heat, and simmer it for 20 to 30 minutes, or until the veggies are soft.

Optional Additions:

If desired, add leafy greens like spinach or kale during the last few minutes of cooking, allowing them to wilt into the soup.

You can also add cooked legumes like lentils or beans for extra protein and fiber, or whole grains like quinoa or barley for added texture and nutrients.

Season to Taste:

Taste the soup and adjust the seasoning as needed, adding more salt, pepper, or herbs to suit your taste preferences.

Serve:
Ladle the Healthy Vegetable Soup into bowls and serve hot. Optionally, garnish with fresh herbs or a drizzle of olive oil before serving.

Storage:
Allow any leftover soup to cool completely before transferring it to an airtight container and refrigerating or freezing for later enjoyment.

Healthy Vegetable Soup is a versatile dish that can be customized based on your dietary preferences and what ingredients you have on hand. It's a delicious and comforting way to incorporate a variety of vegetables into your diet while providing essential nutrients and hydration. Enjoy it as a light meal or starter, or pair it with a salad or crusty bread for a more substantial meal.

Minestrone Soup

Minestrone Soup is a hearty and nutritious
Italian soup packed with a variety of
vegetables, beans, pasta, and flavorful broth.
Here's how to make a healthy version of this
classic dish:

Ingredients
One tablespoon of olive oil
One diced onion, two minced cloves of garlic,
two chopped carrots, two diced celery stalks,
one diced zucchini, one diced yellow squash,
one cup diced green beans, one can (14 oz)
diced tomatoes (low-sodium preferred)
Six cups of vegetable broth low in salt
One tsp of dehydrated oregano
One tsp of dried basil
One-half tsp dried thyme
To taste, add salt and black pepper.
One cup of little pasta, as ditalini or macaroni

One can (15 oz) of washed and drained cannellini beans
For serving, add 2 cups of finely chopped baby spinach or kale and grated Parmesan cheese (optional).

Instructions:

To sauté aromatics, put a large soup pot over medium heat with olive oil. Add the diced onion and garlic, and simmer for 3–4 minutes, or until softened and aromatic.

Add the vegetables: Toss in the green beans, celery, zucchini, yellow squash, and chopped carrots. Cook the vegetables for a further five to seven minutes, or until they begin to soften.

Add the diced tomatoes (together with their juices) and the veggie broth and simmer. Add the basil, thyme, dried oregano, salt, and black pepper and stir. To enable the flavors to mingle, bring the soup to a simmer and cook for around 15 minutes.

Cook Pasta:
While the soup is simmering, cook the pasta separately according to the package instructions until al dente. Drain and set aside.

Add Beans and Greens:
Add the cooked pasta and cannellini beans to the soup pot. Stir in the chopped spinach or kale and let the soup simmer for an additional 5 minutes, or until the greens are wilted and the pasta is heated through.

Taste the soup and add more salt and pepper if necessary to adjust the seasoning. If needed, you can also add extra stock to change the soup's thickness.

To serve, ladle the hot minestrone soup into dishes. For more taste, you can optionally top with grated Parmesan cheese before serving.

Storage: For up to three to four days, keep any leftovers in the refrigerator in an airtight container. Over time, the flavors will intensify, making it even more mouthwatering when reheated.

Minestrone Soup is a nutritious and satisfying meal that's perfect for any time of year. Packed with a variety of vegetables, beans, and pasta, it's a wholesome dish that will keep you warm and full while providing essential nutrients. Enjoy it as a starter, side dish, or even a main course with a slice of crusty bread on the side. Buon !

Lentil and Vegetable Stew

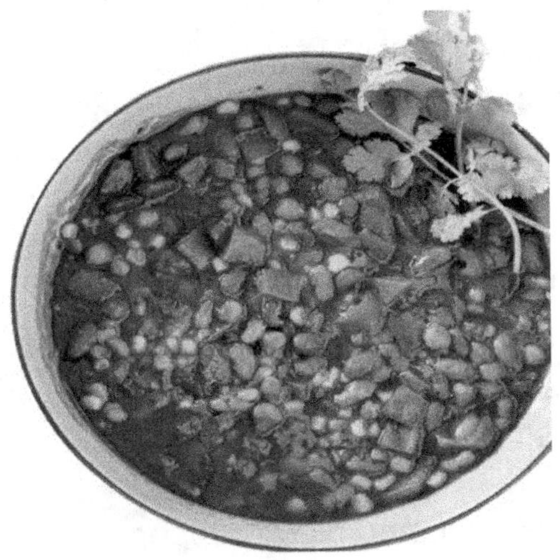

Lentil and Vegetable Stew is a hearty and nutritious dish that combines protein-rich lentils with a variety of vegetables and flavorful broth. Here's how to make it:

Ingredients:
One cup of washed and drained dried lentils,
either brown or green
One tablespoon of olive oil
One onion, chopped, two garlic cloves, minced,
two carrots, chopped, two celery stalks,
chopped, one bell pepper (any color), chopped,
one zucchini, chopped
One cup of canned or fresh diced tomatoes
Four cups vegetable broth with minimal sodium
and 1 teaspoon dried thyme
One tsp of dehydrated rosemary
To taste, add salt and black pepper.
Not required: Use fresh herbs as garnish, like
cilantro or parsley.

Instructions:

Cook Lentils:
In a large pot, combine the rinsed lentils with enough water to cover them by about an inch. Bring to a boil, then reduce heat to medium-low and simmer for 20-25 minutes, or until the lentils are tender but not mushy.
Drain any excess water and set the lentils aside.

In the same pot, warm up some olive oil over medium heat for sautéing aromatics. Add the diced onion and garlic, and simmer for 3–4 minutes, or until softened and aromatic.

Add Vegetables: Add zucchini, bell pepper, celery, and chopped carrots to the saucepan. Cook the vegetables for a further five to seven minutes, or until they begin to soften.

Add the chopped tomatoes, dry thyme, and dried rosemary, and simmer with the broth. After adding the vegetable broth, boil the mixture.

Combine Lentils and Vegetables:
Add the cooked lentils to the pot with the vegetables and broth. Stir to combine, then cover and let the stew simmer for about 15-20 minutes, allowing the flavors to meld together.

Season to Taste: Use salt and black pepper to taste the stew and adjust the seasoning as necessary. If preferred, you can also add extra broth or water to change the stew's thickness.

Serve:
Ladle the Lentil and Vegetable Stew into bowls and garnish with fresh herbs if desired. Serve hot and enjoy!

Optional Additions:
You can customize this stew by adding additional vegetables such as spinach, kale, potatoes, or sweet potatoes.

For extra protein, consider adding cooked chickpeas, black beans, or tofu cubes to the stew.

Feel free to experiment with different herbs and spices to suit your taste preferences, such as cumin, paprika, or bay leaves.

Lentil and Vegetable Stew is a wholesome and satisfying meal that's perfect for chilly days. Packed with fiber, protein, vitamins, and minerals from the lentils and vegetables, it's a nutritious option for lunch or dinner. Enjoy it as a standalone dish or serve it with crusty bread or a side salad for a complete meal.

Butternut Squash Soup

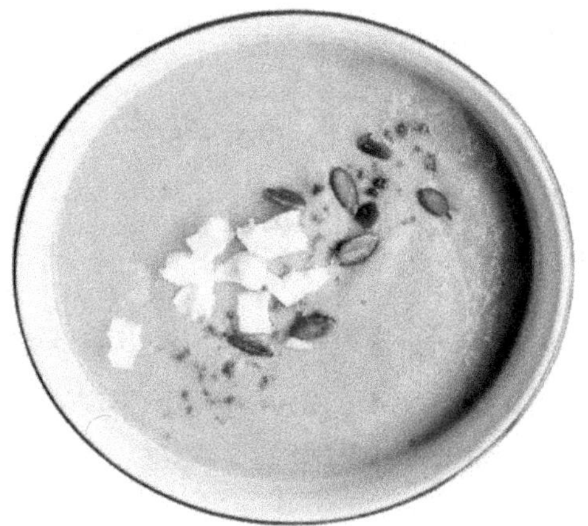

Butternut Squash Soup is a creamy and comforting dish that highlights the sweet and nutty flavor of butternut squash. Here's how to make it:

Ingredients:
One medium butternut squash, roughly four
cups, peeled, seeded, and chopped
1 onion, diced
2 cloves garlic, minced
2 carrots, diced
2 celery stalks, diced
4 cups low-sodium vegetable broth
1 teaspoon dried thyme
1/2 teaspoon ground cinnamon
1/4 teaspoon ground nutmeg
Salt and black pepper to taste
2 tablespoons olive oil or butter
Optional garnish: Greek yogurt or coconut milk,
toasted pumpkin seeds, fresh herbs (such as
parsley or chives).

Instructions:

Preheat Oven:
Preheat your oven to 400°F (200°C).

Roast Butternut Squash: Spread out the chopped squash on a parchment paper-lined baking sheet. Add a drizzle of melted butter or one tablespoon of olive oil, and season with black pepper and salt. For an even coat, toss. Roast the squash for 25 to 30 minutes in a preheated oven, or until it's soft and has a light caramelized color.

To sauté aromatics, put the remaining tablespoon of butter or olive oil in a big pot and heat it over medium heat. Add the celery, carrots, diced onion, and garlic. Simmer for 5 to 7 minutes, or until the veggies are tender, stirring periodically.

Simmer with Broth and Spices: Combine the sautéed vegetables in a pot and add the roasted butternut squash. After adding the low-sodium vegetable broth, whisk everything together.

Add ground nutmeg, ground cinnamon, and dried thyme to the dish. After giving everything a good stir, reduce the heat to a simmer.

Blend Soup:
Using an immersion blender or transferring the soup in batches to a blender, blend until smooth and creamy. Be careful when blending hot liquids.

If the soup is too thick, you can add more vegetable broth or water to reach your desired consistency.

Before serving, taste the soup and add more salt and black pepper if necessary. Mix thoroughly to blend.

Spoon the Butternut Squash Soup into bowls; if preferred, top with toasted pumpkin seeds, fresh herbs, and a dollop of Greek yogurt or coconut milk.

Optional Additions:
For extra creaminess, you can add a splash of coconut milk or cream to the soup before blending.

Add a pinch of cayenne pepper or red pepper flakes for a hint of heat.
Consider incorporating other seasonal spices like ginger or curry powder for additional flavor.

Butternut Squash Soup is a nutritious and satisfying meal that's perfect for cozy nights. Rich in vitamins, minerals, and antioxidants, it's a healthy vegetable recipe that's sure to warm you up from the inside out. Enjoy it as a starter or pair it with a salad or crusty bread for a complete meal.

CHAPTER FOUR

Stir-Fries and Sautes

Stir-fries and sautés are quick and versatile cooking methods that allow you to prepare healthy vegetable recipes with minimal time and effort. Here's an overview of both techniques:

Stir-Fries:

High Heat Cooking: Stir-frying involves cooking vegetables (and often protein) quickly over high heat in a small amount of oil. The high heat helps to retain the vegetables' crispness while sealing in their natural flavors and nutrients.

Versatility: You can use a wide variety of vegetables in stir-fries, including bell peppers, broccoli, carrots, snap peas, mushrooms, onions, and more. This makes it easy to incorporate a diverse range of nutrients into your meals.

Speedy Preparation: Stir-fries are perfect for busy weeknights because they come together quickly. Once you've chopped your vegetables and protein, the cooking process takes only a few minutes.

Healthy Cooking Method: Since stir-frying typically uses minimal oil and short cooking times, it's a healthier cooking method compared to deep-frying or pan-frying. Plus, the abundance of vegetables makes stir-fries rich in vitamins, minerals, and fiber.

Sautés:

Medium to High Heat Cooking: Sautéing involves cooking vegetables (and often aromatics like onions and garlic) over medium to high heat in a skillet or sauté pan with a small amount of oil or butter. The goal is to lightly brown the vegetables while preserving their texture and flavor.

Quick and Simple: Like stir-fries, sautés are quick and easy to prepare, making them perfect for busy weeknights. You can have a flavorful and nutritious meal on the table in a matter of minutes.

Flavor Infusion: Sautéing allows you to develop rich flavors by caramelizing the natural sugars in the vegetables. This adds depth and complexity to your dishes without the need for heavy sauces or seasonings.

Customizable: You can customize sautés based on your preferences and what's in season. Experiment with different combinations of vegetables, herbs, and spices to create your own unique flavor profiles.

Tips for Healthy Stir-Fries and Sautés:

Use Healthy Fats: Opt for heart-healthy fats like olive oil, avocado oil, or coconut oil when cooking stir-fries and sautés.

Load Up on Vegetables: Make vegetables the star of your dish by including a variety of colorful options. Aim to fill at least half of your plate with vegetables for a nutrient-packed meal.

Add Lean Protein: Incorporate lean protein sources like chicken breast, tofu, shrimp, or beans to make your stir-fries and sautés more filling and balanced.

Mindful Seasoning: Use herbs, spices, and citrus zest to add flavor to your dishes without relying on excess salt or sugar.

Pair with Whole Grains: Serve your stir-fries and sautés with whole grains like brown rice, quinoa, or whole wheat noodles for added fiber and nutrients.

By mastering the techniques of stir-frying and sautéing, you can create delicious and healthy vegetable recipes that are both satisfying and nutritious. Experiment with different ingredients and flavor combinations to keep your meals exciting and enjoyable.

Vegetable Stir-Fry with Brown Rice

Vegetable Stir-Fry with Brown Rice is a delicious and nutritious dish that combines colorful vegetables with whole grains for a satisfying meal. Here's how to make it:

Ingredients:
For the Stir-Fry:
2 cups mixed vegetables (such as bell peppers, broccoli, carrots, snap peas, mushrooms, onions)
2 tablespoons olive oil or sesame oil
2 cloves garlic, minced
1 tablespoon fresh ginger, grated or minced
1 tablespoon low-sodium soy sauce or tamari
1 tablespoon rice vinegar or lime juice
Optional: 1 teaspoon chili garlic sauce or sriracha for heat
Salt and black pepper to taste.

For the Brown Rice:
1 cup brown rice
2 cups water or vegetable broth
Pinch of salt
Optional Garnishes:
Sliced green onions
Toasted sesame seeds
Chopped cilantro or parsley.

Instructions:

For the Brown Rice:
Rinse Rice: Rinse the brown rice under cold water until the water runs clear to remove excess starch.

Cook Rice: Place the washed brown rice, water or vegetable broth, and a small amount of salt in a medium pot. Over high heat, bring to a boil.

After that, lower the heat to a simmer, cover, and cook for 40 to 45 minutes, or until the rice is soft and the liquid has been absorbed.Take it off the heat and leave it covered for five minutes. Use a fork to fluff before serving.

For the Vegetable Stir-Fry:

Prepare Vegetables: Wash and chop the mixed vegetables into bite-sized pieces. Keep the vegetables separated according to their cooking times (e.g., harder vegetables like carrots and broccoli will take longer to cook than softer vegetables like bell peppers and snap peas).

Heat Oil: Heat olive oil or sesame oil in a large skillet or wok over medium-high heat.

Sauté Aromatics: Add minced garlic and grated ginger to the hot oil and stir-fry for about 30 seconds, or until fragrant.

Add Vegetables: Add the harder vegetables to the skillet first (such as carrots and broccoli) and stir-fry for 2-3 minutes. Then add the remaining vegetables and continue to stir-fry for another 2-3 minutes, or until all the vegetables are tender-crisp.

To season, combine soy sauce, tamari, rice vinegar, lime juice, and optional chili garlic sauce or sriracha in a small bowl. After pouring the sauce over the veggies, toss to ensure even coating. To taste, add salt and black pepper for seasoning.

Serve: Divide the cooked brown rice among serving bowls and top with the vegetable stir-fry. Garnish with sliced green onions, toasted sesame seeds, and chopped cilantro or parsley if desired.

Tips:
Customize the stir-fry with your favorite vegetables and adjust the seasoning to suit your taste preferences.
For added protein, toss in some cooked tofu, chicken, shrimp, or edamame.
Make extra brown rice and store it in the refrigerator for quick and easy meal prep.

Garlic and Ginger Broccoli Stir-Fry

Garlic and Ginger Broccoli Stir-Fry is a flavorful and nutritious dish that highlights the natural sweetness of broccoli with the aromatic and zesty flavors of garlic and ginger. Here's how to make it:

Ingredients:
1 head of broccoli, cut into florets
2 tablespoons olive oil or sesame oil
3 cloves garlic, minced
1 tablespoon fresh ginger, grated or minced
2 tablespoons low-sodium soy sauce or tamari
1 tablespoon rice vinegar or lime juice
1 teaspoon of honey or maple syrup is optional but adds a touch of sweetness

Optional: Red pepper flakes or chili garlic sauce for heat
Salt and black pepper to taste
Optional garnish: Sliced green onions, toasted sesame seeds.

Instructions:
Prepare Broccoli: Wash the broccoli under cold water and cut it into bite-sized florets. Trim and discard the tough ends of the broccoli stalks.

Blanch Broccoli (Optional): If you prefer your broccoli to be tender-crisp, you can blanch it in boiling water for 1-2 minutes, then immediately transfer it to a bowl of ice water to stop the cooking process. Drain and set aside.

Heat Oil: Heat olive oil or sesame oil in a large skillet or wok over medium-high heat.

Sauté Aromatics: Add minced garlic and grated ginger to the hot oil and stir-fry for about 30 seconds, or until fragrant.

Stir-Fry Broccoli: Add the broccoli florets to the skillet and stir-fry for 3-4 minutes, or until the broccoli is tender but still vibrant green.

Make Sauce: In a small bowl, mix together low-sodium soy sauce or tamari, rice vinegar or lime juice, and optional honey or maple syrup. Pour the sauce over the broccoli and toss to coat evenly.

Season and Serve: Add salt and black pepper to taste while seasoning the stir-fried broccoli. For more spice, top with chili garlic sauce or red pepper flakes, if using. If preferred, garnish with toasted sesame seeds and sliced green onions.

Tips:
Adjust the amount of garlic and ginger
according to your taste preferences. You can
add more for a stronger flavor or reduce the
amount for a milder taste.

Customize the stir-fry by adding other
vegetables such as bell peppers, snap peas,
carrots, or mushrooms.
Serve the Garlic and Ginger Broccoli Stir-Fry
as a side dish or as a main course with cooked
rice, quinoa, or noodles.

Mushroom and Bell Pepper Saute

Mushroom and Bell Pepper Sauté is a simple yet flavorful dish that brings together the earthy richness of mushrooms with the sweet crunchiness of bell peppers. Here's how to make it:

Ingredients:
2 cups mushrooms, sliced (such as button mushrooms, cremini, or shiitake)
1 bell pepper (any color), thinly sliced
2 cloves garlic, minced
2 tablespoons olive oil or butter
Salt and black pepper to taste
Optional: Fresh herbs (such as thyme or parsley) for garnish.

Instructions:

Prepare Ingredients: Wash the mushrooms to remove any dirt, then slice them thinly. Thinly slice the bell pepper as well. Mince the garlic cloves.

Sauté Mushrooms: Heat olive oil or butter in a large skillet over medium heat. Add the sliced mushrooms to the skillet and cook, stirring occasionally, for about 5-7 minutes, or until the mushrooms are golden brown and tender.

Add Bell Pepper: Once the mushrooms are cooked, add the sliced bell pepper to the skillet. Cook, stirring occasionally, for an additional 3-4 minutes, or until the bell pepper is tender-crisp.

Add Garlic: Add the minced garlic to the skillet and cook for another 1-2 minutes, or until the garlic is fragrant. Be careful not to burn the garlic.

Season: Season the mushroom and bell pepper sauté with salt and black pepper to taste. Stir well to combine and allow the flavors to meld together.

Garnish and Serve: Garnish the sauté with fresh herbs like thyme or parsley if desired. Serve hot as a side dish or as a topping for cooked grains, pasta, or toast.

Tips:
Feel free to customize the sauté by adding other vegetables such as onions, zucchini, or spinach.

For extra flavor, you can add a splash of balsamic vinegar or soy sauce to the skillet while cooking.

Serve the Mushroom and Bell Pepper Sauté as a versatile side dish, or incorporate it into other dishes like omelets, sandwiches, wraps, or grain bowls.

Tofu and Vegetable Stir-Fry

A tasty sauce is stir-fried together with a variety of colorful veggies and protein-rich tofu to create a dish that is both gratifying and nutritious. This is how to prepare it:

Ingredients:

For the Stir-Fry:
1 block (14-16 oz) extra-firm tofu, pressed and cubed
2 tablespoons soy sauce or tamari
1 tablespoon cornstarch
2 tablespoons sesame oil or olive oil
3 cloves garlic, minced
1 tablespoon fresh ginger, grated or minced
1 bell pepper (any color), thinly sliced
1 cup broccoli florets
1 carrot, julienned or thinly sliced
One cup of clipped snap peas or snow peas
Optional: Other vegetables such as

mushrooms, baby corn, or water chestnuts
Salt and black pepper to taste
For the Sauce:
1/4 cup low-sodium soy sauce or tamari
2 tablespoons rice vinegar or lime juice
1 tablespoon maple syrup or honey
1 teaspoon cornstarch
Optional: Red pepper flakes for heat
Optional Garnishes:
Sliced green onions
Toasted sesame seeds
Chopped cilantro or parsley.

Instructions:

Tofu preparation: Press the tofu to squeeze off extra liquid. After cutting the pressed tofu into cubes, throw them in a mixture of 1 tablespoon cornstarch, 2 tablespoons soy sauce, or tamari, and stir until well coated.

To make the sauce, combine 1/4 cup soy sauce or tamari, 1 teaspoon cornstarch, rice vinegar or lime juice, and maple syrup or honey in a small bowl. Add a small amount of red pepper flakes for spiciness if preferred.

Stir-Fry Tofu: In a large skillet or wok over medium-high heat, heat 1 tablespoon of sesame oil or olive oil. Add the tofu cubes and cook, stirring regularly, for 5 to 7 minutes, or until golden brown and crispy all over. After taking the tofu out of the skillet, set it aside.

Add the last tablespoon of oil to the same skillet and sauté aromatics. Cook the grated ginger and minced garlic for 30 seconds or until fragrant.

Add Vegetables: Add the sliced bell pepper, broccoli florets, julienned carrot, and snap peas to the skillet. Stir-fry for 4-5 minutes, or until the vegetables are tender-crisp.

Tofu and Sauce Combination: Add the cooked tofu back to the skillet along with the veggies. Drizzle the tofu and veggies with the sauce, then mix to ensure even coating. Simmer for a further one to two minutes, or until the sauce has somewhat thickened.

Season and Serve: Season the tofu and vegetable stir-fry with salt and black pepper to taste. Garnish with sliced green onions, toasted sesame seeds, and chopped cilantro or parsley if desired.

Tips:

For extra flavor, marinate the tofu cubes in the soy sauce or tamari mixture for 30 minutes to 1 hour before cooking.

Feel free to customize the stir-fry with your favorite vegetables or add-ins such as mushrooms, baby corn, or water chestnuts.

Serve the tofu and vegetable stir-fry over cooked brown rice, quinoa, or noodles for a complete and satisfying meal.

CHAPTER FIVE

Roasted Vegetables

Roasted vegetables are a simple and delicious way to prepare a wide variety of vegetables, bringing out their natural sweetness and enhancing their flavor through caramelization. Here's how to make roasted vegetables as a part of healthy vegetable recipes:

Ingredients:
Assorted vegetables (such as carrots, bell peppers, broccoli, cauliflower, zucchini, sweet potatoes, Brussels sprouts, cherry tomatoes, etc.)
Olive oil or avocado oil
Salt and pepper
Optional: Herbs and spices (such as garlic powder, onion powder, paprika, thyme, rosemary, etc.).

Instructions:

Preheat Oven: Preheat your oven to 425°F (220°C) and line a baking sheet with parchment paper or aluminum foil for easy cleanup.

Prepare Vegetables: Wash and dry your vegetables thoroughly. Chop them into bite-sized pieces, ensuring they are relatively uniform in size for even cooking.

Apply Oil: Transfer the diced veggies into a big basin. Use enough olive or avocado oil to lightly coat all the vegetables when you drizzle it over them. Make sure the veggies are well covered by giving them a good toss.

To season, add a dash of salt and pepper to the vegetables. For added taste, you can also add other herbs and spices like paprika, thyme, rosemary, onion powder, and garlic powder.

Roast: Spread the seasoned vegetables in a single layer on the prepared baking sheet, making sure they are not overcrowded. This allows them to roast evenly and develop a nice caramelized exterior.

Bake: Place the baking sheet in the preheated oven and roast the vegetables for 20-25 minutes, stirring halfway through, or until they are tender and golden brown.

Serve: Once roasted to perfection, remove the vegetables from the oven and transfer them to a serving dish. Serve hot as a side dish or incorporate them into other recipes, such as salads, grain bowls, wraps, or pasta dishes.

Tips:
Customize your roasted vegetables based on your preferences and what's in season. Experiment with different combinations of vegetables and herbs/spices for variety.

To prevent the vegetables from sticking to the baking sheet, make sure they are well-coated with oil and spread them out evenly in a single layer.

For even roasting, avoid overcrowding the baking sheet. If necessary, use multiple baking sheets or roast the vegetables in batches.

Leftover roasted vegetables can be stored in an airtight container in the refrigerator for up to 3-4 days. They can be reheated in the oven or microwave for a quick and convenient meal.

Oven Roasted-Brussels Sprouts

Oven-roasted Brussels sprouts are a delightful and nutritious dish that transforms these cruciferous vegetables into crispy, caramelized bites bursting with flavor. Here's how to make them:

Ingredients:
1 lb Brussels sprouts, trimmed and halved
2 tablespoons olive oil
Salt and black pepper to taste
Optional: Balsamic glaze, grated Parmesan cheese, or crispy bacon bits for serving.

Instructions:

Preheat Oven: Preheat your oven to 400°F (200°C) and line a baking sheet with parchment paper or aluminum foil.

To prepare Brussels sprouts, give them a good wash and cut off the tough ends. To cook them more quickly and evenly, cut them in half lengthwise.

Coat with Oil: Transfer the Brussels sprouts, cut in half, to a big bowl. Make sure they are evenly coated by drizzling them with olive oil. Toss well to evenly distribute the oil over each sprout.

To season, add a dash of black pepper and salt to the Brussels sprouts. For added flavor, you can also add other seasonings such smoked paprika, onion powder, and garlic powder.

Roast: Spread the seasoned Brussels sprouts in a single layer on the prepared baking sheet, cut side down. This allows them to caramelize and develop a crispy exterior.

Bake: For 20 to 25 minutes, or until golden brown and fork-tender, place the baking sheet in the preheated oven and roast the Brussels sprouts. To guarantee uniform browning, stir halfway during cooking.

Serve: Once roasted to perfection, remove the Brussels sprouts from the oven and transfer them to a serving dish. Drizzle with balsamic glaze, sprinkle with grated Parmesan cheese, or top with crispy bacon bits if desired.

Tips:
Choose Brussels sprouts that are firm, bright green, and similar in size for even cooking.

Trim any discolored or damaged outer leaves and slice off the tough ends before roasting.

For extra crispiness, you can increase the oven temperature to 425°F (220°C) and roast for a shorter time, around 15-20 minutes.

For up to three to four days, leftover roasted Brussels sprouts can be kept in the refrigerator in an airtight container. Before serving, reheat them in the microwave or oven.

Brussels sprouts are a tasty and wholesome side dish that works well for any occasion when baked in the oven. Their enticing flavor and crispy texture make them popular as a complement to weeknight dinners or as a side dish for holidays.

Honey Glazed Carrots

Honey glazed carrots are a delightful and nutritious dish that combines the natural sweetness of carrots with a sticky, caramelized glaze made from honey. Here's how to make them:

Ingredients:
1 lb carrots, peeled and sliced into rounds or sticks
2 tablespoons unsalted butter or olive oil
2 tablespoons honey
Salt and black pepper to taste
Garnish with optional fresh herbs, such thyme or parsley.

Instructions:

Prepare Carrots: Peel the carrots and slice them into rounds or sticks, depending on your preference.

Steam Carrots (Optional): If desired, you can steam the carrots for a few minutes to partially cook them and make them more tender.

Cook the Carrots: Melt the butter in a large skillet or saucepan over medium heat. When the carrots begin to soften, add them to the skillet with the slices and cook, stirring now and again, for about five to seven minutes.

Add Honey: Drizzle the honey over the cooked carrots in the skillet. Stir well to coat the carrots evenly with the honey glaze.

Caramelize: Continue to cook the carrots, stirring occasionally, for another 5-7 minutes, or until they are caramelized and glazed, and the honey thickens slightly.

Season: Season the honey glazed carrots with salt and black pepper to taste. Adjust the seasoning if needed.

Garnish and Serve: Transfer the honey glazed carrots to a serving dish and garnish with fresh herbs like parsley or thyme if desired. Serve hot as a side dish or accompaniment to your favorite main course.

Tips:
Choose fresh, firm carrots for the best flavor and texture.

You can customize the honey glaze by adding other ingredients such as balsamic vinegar, orange juice, or spices like cinnamon or ginger.

Be careful not to overcook the carrots, as they should still have a slight crunch to them after caramelizing.

You may keep leftover honey-glazed carrots in the fridge for up to three to four days if you put them in an airtight container.

Before serving, reheat them in the stovetop or microwave.

A tasty and eye-catching side dish that works well for any occasion, from weeknight dinners to holiday feasts, is honey-glazed carrots. They will appeal to both children and adults due to their inherent sweetness and glossy finish.

Parmesan Roasted Cauliflower

Parmesan roasted cauliflower is a flavorful and nutritious dish that elevates the humble cauliflower to new heights by roasting it to perfection with a crispy Parmesan crust. Here's how to make it:

Ingredients:
1 head cauliflower, cut into florets
2 tablespoons olive oil
1/4 cup grated Parmesan cheese
1 teaspoon garlic powder
1/2 teaspoon onion powder
1/2 teaspoon smoked paprika (optional)
Salt and black pepper to taste
Optional: Chopped fresh parsley or thyme for garnish.

Instructions:

Preheat Oven: Preheat your oven to 425°F (220°C) and line a baking sheet with parchment paper or aluminum foil for easy cleanup.

Prepare Cauliflower: Wash the cauliflower and cut it into florets, ensuring they are relatively uniform in size for even cooking.

Toss the cauliflower florets in a big dish and coat with oil. To ensure even coating, drizzle with olive oil and toss thoroughly.

To season, combine the shredded Parmesan cheese, onion powder, garlic powder, and smoked paprika (if using) in a small bowl. After uniformly coating the cauliflower florets, sprinkle the seasoning mixture on top and toss. To taste, add salt and black pepper for seasoning.

Roast: Spread the seasoned cauliflower florets in a single layer on the prepared baking sheet. This allows them to roast evenly and develop a crispy Parmesan crust.

Bake: Roast the cauliflower for 20 to 25 minutes, or until it is soft and golden brown when poked with a fork, after placing the baking sheet in the preheated oven. To guarantee uniform browning, stir halfway during cooking.

Garnish and Serve: Once roasted to perfection, remove the cauliflower from the oven and transfer it to a serving dish. Garnish with chopped fresh parsley or thyme if desired. Serve hot as a side dish or appetizer.

Tips:
Customize the seasoning to suit your taste preferences. You can experiment with different herbs and spices, such as rosemary, thyme, or cayenne pepper, for added flavor.

You can broil the cauliflower for the final two to three minutes of cooking for even more crispiness.

Leftover Parmesan roasted cauliflower can be stored in an airtight container in the refrigerator for up to 3-4 days. Reheat it in the oven or toaster oven before serving.

Parmesan roasted cauliflower is a delicious and healthy vegetable dish that's perfect for any occasion. With its crispy texture and savory Parmesan flavor, it's sure to be a hit with your family and friends.

Roasted Root Vegetables

Roasted root vegetables are a delicious and nutritious dish that brings out the natural sweetness and flavors of hearty vegetables like carrots, potatoes, parsnips, and beets. This simple cooking method enhances the vegetables' taste and texture, making them tender on the inside and crispy on the outside. Here's how to make roasted root vegetables:

Ingredients:
Assorted root vegetables (such as carrots, potatoes, sweet potatoes, parsnips, beets, turnips, rutabagas)
Olive oil or vegetable oil
Salt and black pepper
Optional: Herbs and spices (such as rosemary, thyme, garlic powder, paprika).

Instructions:

Preheat Oven: Preheat your oven to 425°F (220°C) and line a baking sheet with parchment paper or aluminum foil for easy cleanup.

Prepare Vegetables: Wash and peel the root vegetables as needed. Cut them into evenly sized pieces, about 1-inch cubes or slices, to ensure even cooking.

Coat with Oil: Place the chopped root vegetables in a large bowl. Drizzle with olive oil or vegetable oil, using enough to lightly coat all the vegetables. Toss well to ensure they are evenly coated with oil.

Season: Sprinkle the vegetables with salt and black pepper to taste. You can also add herbs and spices like rosemary, thyme, garlic powder, or paprika for extra flavor.

Roast: Arrange the seasoned root vegetables on the ready baking sheet in a single layer. This makes it possible for them to roast evenly and get a crispy outside.

Bake: Place the baking sheet in the preheated oven and roast the vegetables for 30-40 minutes, or until they are tender and golden brown, stirring halfway through cooking for even browning.

Serve: Once roasted to perfection, remove the root vegetables from the oven and transfer them to a serving dish. Serve hot as a side dish or as a main course with grains or protein.

Tips:
Mix and match your favorite root vegetables to create a colorful and flavorful dish. Consider including carrots, potatoes, sweet potatoes, parsnips, beets, turnips, or rutabagas.

Avoid packing the baking sheet too full as this may hinder the vegetables from roasting in an even manner. If necessary, roast the vegetables in batches or use several baking sheets.

For extra caramelization, you can drizzle the vegetables with a bit of honey or maple syrup before roasting.

Leftover roasted root vegetables can be stored in an airtight container in the refrigerator for up to 3-4 days. Reheat them in the oven or toaster oven before serving.

A tasty and adaptable recipe, roasted root vegetables are ideal for weeknight dinners as well as holiday feasts. They're going to quickly become a staple in your repertoire of healthy vegetable recipes because of their mouthwatering flavor and substantial texture.

CHAPTER SIX

Vegetable Side Dishes

Vegetable side dishes are flavorful accompaniments to the main course that showcase the natural goodness of vegetables. They complement the flavors and textures of the main dish, adding color, nutrients, and variety to the meal. Here are some key points about vegetable side dishes:

Nutrient-Rich: Vegetables are packed with essential vitamins, minerals, and antioxidants that contribute to overall health and well-being. Incorporating a variety of vegetables into side dishes ensures a diverse range of nutrients in your diet.

Versatility: Vegetable side dishes can be prepared in various ways, including roasting, steaming, sautéing, grilling, or serving raw in salads. This versatility allows you to create dishes that suit your taste preferences and dietary needs.

Enhanced Flavor: Vegetables can be seasoned and cooked in a variety of ways to enhance their natural flavors. Adding herbs, spices, garlic, onions, citrus zest, or a drizzle of olive oil can elevate the taste of vegetables and make them more appealing.

Colorful Presentation: Vegetables come in a rainbow of colors, from vibrant greens and reds to rich oranges and purples. Incorporating a variety of colorful vegetables into side dishes not only adds visual appeal to the meal but also indicates a diverse range of nutrients.

Balanced Meal: Including vegetable side dishes in your meal helps create a balanced plate by providing fiber, vitamins, and minerals alongside proteins and carbohydrates. Aim to fill at least half of your plate with vegetables for a nutritious and satisfying meal.

Customizable: Vegetable side dishes can be easily customized based on personal preferences, dietary restrictions, and seasonal availability. You can mix and match different vegetables, experiment with cooking methods, and adjust seasonings to create unique and delicious dishes.

Health Benefits: Consuming a diet rich in vegetables has been associated with numerous health benefits, including reduced risk of chronic diseases such as heart disease, diabetes, and certain types of cancer. Vegetable side dishes contribute to overall health and well-being when included as part of a balanced diet.

Steamed Broccoli with Lemon Butter Sauce

Steamed broccoli with lemon butter sauce is a simple yet delicious and healthy vegetable recipe that combines tender steamed broccoli florets with a zesty and flavorful lemon butter sauce. Here's how to make it:

Ingredients:
1 lb broccoli florets
2 tablespoons unsalted butter
2 cloves garlic, minced
Zest of 1 lemon
Juice of 1 lemon
Salt and black pepper to taste
Optional: Red pepper flakes for heat
Garnish options include grated Parmesan cheese or freshly chopped parsley.

Instructions:

Steam Broccoli: Place the broccoli florets in a steamer basket set over a pot of boiling water. Cover and steam for 5-7 minutes, or until the broccoli is tender but still vibrant green. Remove from heat and transfer the steamed broccoli to a serving dish.

Prepare Lemon Butter Sauce: In a small saucepan, melt the unsalted butter over medium heat. Add the minced garlic and sauté for 1-2 minutes, or until fragrant.

Add Lemon Zest and Juice: Add the lemon zest and juice to the saucepan with the melted butter and garlic. Stir well to combine. If desired, add a pinch of red pepper flakes for a hint of heat.

Season: Season the lemon butter sauce with salt and black pepper to taste. Adjust the seasoning as needed.

Pour Sauce Over Broccoli: Pour the lemon butter sauce over the steamed broccoli in the serving dish. Toss gently to coat the broccoli evenly with the sauce.

Garnish and Serve: Garnish the steamed broccoli with fresh chopped parsley or grated Parmesan cheese if desired. Serve hot as a side dish or accompaniment to your favorite main course.

Tips

Broccoli can turn mushy and lose its brilliant color if it is overcooked, so proceed with caution. For optimal texture, steam it just till tender-crisp.

To suit your taste, dilute or increase the amount of lemon zest and juice. You can add extra zest or juice for a more intense lemon flavor.

Feel free to customize the sauce with additional ingredients such as minced shallots, fresh herbs like thyme or basil, or a splash of white wine for added depth of flavor.

For up to two or three days, leftover steamed broccoli with lemon butter sauce can be kept in the refrigerator in an airtight container. Before serving, give it a quick reheat in the microwave or on the stove.

From weeknight dinners to holiday feasts, steamed broccoli with lemon butter sauce is a light and refreshing vegetable dish that works well for any occasion. It's guaranteed to be a success with your family and friends thanks to its vivid colors and flavors.

Grilled Asparagus with Balsamic Glaze

Grilled asparagus with balsamic glaze is a flavorful and nutritious vegetable dish that combines the smoky char of grilled asparagus with the tangy sweetness of balsamic glaze. Here's how to make it:

Ingredients:

1 lb asparagus spears, trimmed
1-2 tablespoons olive oil
Salt and black pepper to taste
Balsamic glaze (store-bought or homemade)
Garnish options include chopped fresh herbs (like thyme or parsley) and grated Parmesan cheese.

Instructions:

Preheat Grill: Preheat your grill to medium-high heat, around 400°F (200°C).

To prepare the asparagus, wash it and cut off the rough ends. Then use a paper towel to pat them dry.

Dredge in Oil: Transfer the clipped asparagus spears to a big basin. To ensure even coating, drizzle with olive oil and toss thoroughly.

To season, add a dash of black pepper and salt to the asparagus. Toss once more to make sure all of the seasoning is included.

Grill Asparagus: Place the seasoned asparagus spears directly on the preheated grill. Grill for 4-6 minutes, turning occasionally, or until the asparagus is tender and slightly charred.

Drizzle with Balsamic Glaze: Once the asparagus is grilled to perfection, transfer it to a serving platter. Drizzle with balsamic glaze, using as much or as little as desired.

Garnish and Serve: Garnish the grilled asparagus with grated Parmesan cheese and chopped fresh herbs if desired. Serve hot as a side dish or appetizer.

Tips:
Choose medium to thick asparagus spears for grilling, as they hold up better on the grill and develop a nice char without becoming too limp.

Be sure to monitor the asparagus closely while grilling to prevent it from overcooking and becoming mushy.

If you don't have access to an outdoor grill, you can also grill the asparagus indoors on a grill pan or under the broiler in the oven.

Feel free to customize the dish by adding other seasonings or toppings, such as minced garlic, lemon zest, or toasted nuts.

Leftover grilled asparagus can be stored in an airtight container in the refrigerator for up to 2-3 days. Reheat gently in the microwave or enjoy the cold in salads or sandwiches.

Grilled asparagus with balsamic glaze is a simple yet elegant dish that's perfect for summer cookouts, BBQs, or any time you're craving a delicious and healthy vegetable side. With its bold flavors and vibrant colors, it's sure to be a hit with your family and friends.

Sauteed Green Beans with Almonds

Sauteed green beans with almonds is a flavorful and nutritious vegetable dish that combines crisp-tender green beans with crunchy toasted almonds for a delightful texture contrast. Here's how to make it:

Ingredients:
1 lb green beans, trimmed
2 tablespoons olive oil or butter
2 cloves garlic, minced
1/4 cup sliced almonds
Salt and black pepper to taste
Optional: Lemon zest or juice for added flavor
Optional garnish: Chopped fresh parsley or grated Parmesan cheese.

Instructions:

Prepare Green Beans: Wash the green beans thoroughly and trim off the stem ends. If the beans are long, you can cut them in half for easier cooking.

Toast Almonds: Toast the almond slices, tossing regularly to avoid burning, in a dry skillet over medium heat until aromatic and golden brown. Once on a platter, remove and reserve the roasted almonds.

Saute Garlic: In the same skillet, heat the olive oil or butter over medium heat. Add the minced garlic and sauté for 1-2 minutes, or until fragrant.

Add Green Beans: Add the trimmed green beans to the skillet with the sautéed garlic. Cook, stirring occasionally, for 5-7 minutes, or until the green beans are crisp-tender and bright green.

Season: Season the sautéed green beans with salt and black pepper to taste. You can also add a sprinkle of lemon zest or a squeeze of lemon juice for a bright, citrusy flavor.

Add Almonds: Stir in the toasted almonds, reserving a few for garnish if desired. Toss well to combine and evenly distribute the almonds throughout the green beans.

Garnish and Serve: Spoon the almond-studded sautéed green beans onto a platter. If preferred, garnish with grated Parmesan cheese or chopped fresh parsley. Serve hot as an appetizer or side dish to your preferred entrée.

Tips:
Be careful not to overcook the green beans, as they should be tender but still have a slight crunch to them.

Customize the dish by adding other seasonings or ingredients such as red pepper flakes, shallots, or balsamic vinegar for extra flavor.

If you prefer softer green beans, you can cover the skillet with a lid while cooking to steam them slightly.

For up to two or three days, leftover sautéed green beans with almonds can be kept in the refrigerator in an airtight container. Before serving, reheat gently in the microwave or on the stovetop.

Simple yet elegant, sauteed green beans with almonds make a great meal for weeknight dinners or holiday feasts alike. It is certain to be a big hit with your family and friends thanks to its bright colors, crispy texture, and mouthwatering flavor.

Mashed Sweet Potatoes

Mashed sweet potatoes are a delicious and nutritious side dish that offers a flavorful twist on traditional mashed potatoes. Here's how to make them:

Ingredients:
Two pounds of peeled and chunked sweet potatoes
2–3 teaspoons of olive oil or unsalted butter
1/4 cup of optional vegetarian broth or milk
To taste, add salt and black pepper.
For more taste, feel free to add honey, cinnamon, nutmeg, maple syrup, or other spices.

Instructions:
Cook Sweet Potatoes: Place the peeled and chopped sweet potatoes in a large pot and cover them with water. Bring the water to a boil, then reduce the heat to medium-low and simmer the sweet potatoes for 15-20 minutes, or until they are fork-tender.

Drain and Mash: Once the sweet potatoes are cooked, drain them well and transfer them to a large mixing bowl. Use a potato masher or fork to mash the sweet potatoes until smooth and creamy.

Add Butter: Add the unsalted butter or olive oil to the mashed sweet potatoes. Mix well until the butter is melted and fully incorporated into the mixture.

Adjust Consistency: If desired, add milk or vegetable broth to the mashed sweet potatoes to achieve your desired consistency. Start with a small amount and add more as needed until you reach the desired creaminess.

Season: Season the mashed sweet potatoes with salt and black pepper to taste. You can also add additional flavorings such as maple syrup, honey, cinnamon, nutmeg, or other spices to taste.

Serve: Transfer the mashed sweet potatoes to a serving dish and garnish with a sprinkle of black pepper or a drizzle of melted butter, if desired. Serve hot as a side dish alongside your favorite main course.

Tips:
For consistent cooking, select sweet potatoes with similar sizes.
To prevent mushy mashed potatoes, make sure the cooked sweet potatoes are thoroughly drained.

Add your preferred herbs and flavorings to the mashed sweet potatoes to make it your own.

Sweet potato mash leftovers can be kept in the fridge for up to three to four days when kept in an airtight container. Before serving, give them a quick reheat in the microwave or on the stove.

CHAPTER SEVEN

Veggie Packed Main Courses

Veggie-packed main courses are hearty and nutritious dishes where vegetables play a central role as the main ingredient, providing flavor, texture, and essential nutrients. These dishes are not only delicious but also satisfying, making them suitable for vegetarians, vegans, or anyone looking to incorporate more vegetables into their diet. Here are some key points about veggie-packed main courses:

Nutrient-Rich: Vegetables are rich in vitamins, minerals, fiber, and antioxidants, making them an important part of a balanced diet. By including a variety of vegetables in main courses, you can boost the nutritional value of the meal and support overall health and well-being.

Versatility: Vegetables come in a wide range of flavors, textures, and colors, allowing for endless creativity in the kitchen. From leafy greens and cruciferous vegetables to root vegetables and legumes, there are countless options to choose from when creating veggie-packed main courses.

Satiety: Vegetables are naturally low in calories and high in fiber, which can help promote feelings of fullness and satisfaction. By incorporating plenty of vegetables into main courses, you can create hearty and filling meals without relying heavily on meat or other high-calorie ingredients.

Flavor Enhancement: Vegetables add depth and complexity to main courses, enhancing the overall flavor profile of the dish. Whether roasted, sautéed, grilled, or steamed, vegetables can bring a burst of freshness and vitality to any meal.

Variety: Veggie-packed main courses offer a wide range of culinary possibilities, from comforting stews and casseroles to vibrant salads and stir-fries. Whether you're craving something cozy and comforting or light and refreshing, there's a veggie-packed main course to suit every taste and occasion.

Health Benefits: Consuming a diet rich in vegetables has been associated with numerous health benefits, including reduced risk of chronic diseases such as heart disease, diabetes, and certain types of cancer. Veggie-packed main courses provide an easy and delicious way to incorporate more vegetables into your diet and support overall health.

Environmental Sustainability: Choosing vegetable-based main courses can also have positive environmental impacts by reducing the demand for animal products and lowering greenhouse gas emissions associated with livestock farming.

By incorporating more vegetables into your diet, you can contribute to a more sustainable food system.

Overall, veggie-packed main courses are a delicious and nutritious way to enjoy the abundance of flavors and textures that vegetables have to offer. Whether you're cooking for yourself, your family, or guests, these dishes are sure to impress with their versatility, flavor, and health benefits.

Zucchini Noodles with Pesto

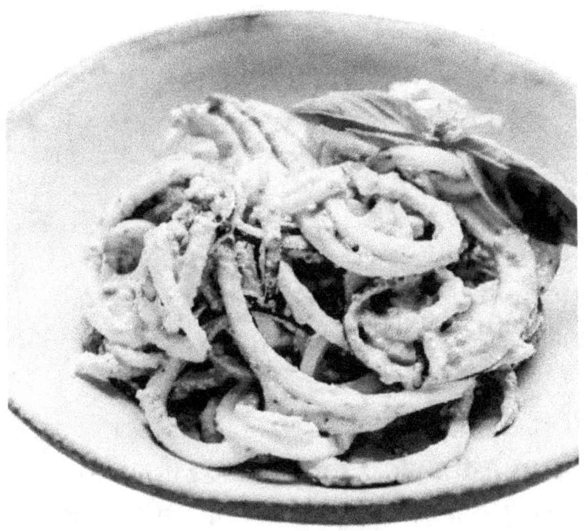

Zucchini noodles with pesto is a light, flavorful, and healthy vegetable recipe that substitutes traditional pasta with spiralized zucchini noodles, or "zoodles," and combines them with a vibrant and aromatic pesto sauce. Here's how to make it:

Ingredients:
4 medium zucchini
1 cup fresh basil leaves
1/4 cup pine nuts or walnuts, toasted
1/4 cup grated Parmesan cheese (optional)
2 cloves garlic
1/4 cup extra-virgin olive oil
Salt and black pepper to taste
Optional toppings: Cherry tomatoes, sliced olives, grilled chicken, or shrimp.

Instructions:
Prepare Zucchini Noodles: Using a spiralizer or vegetable peeler, create zucchini noodles by spiralizing or thinly slicing the zucchini lengthwise. Set the zucchini noodles aside.

To prepare the Pesto Sauce, place the fresh basil leaves, toasted pine nuts or walnuts, grated Parmesan cheese (if desired), garlic cloves, and a dash of black pepper and salt in a food processor or blender. The components should be minced finely after pulsing.

Olive Oil Addition: While the food processor or blender is operating, gradually pour in the extra-virgin olive oil until the pesto sauce has the consistency you want. Blend until smooth, scraping down the sides of the bowl as necessary.

Taste and Adjust: Taste the pesto sauce and adjust the seasoning as needed, adding more salt, pepper, or Parmesan cheese to suit your taste preferences.

Cook Zucchini Noodles: Heat a large skillet over medium heat. Add the zucchini noodles to the skillet and cook for 2-3 minutes, tossing gently with tongs, until the noodles are just tender but still crisp.

Combine with Pesto: Add the pesto sauce to the skillet with the cooked zucchini noodles. Toss well to coat the noodles evenly with the pesto sauce.

Serve: Transfer the zucchini noodles with pesto to serving plates or bowls. Garnish with additional grated Parmesan cheese, toasted pine nuts or walnuts, and optional toppings such as cherry tomatoes, sliced olives, grilled chicken, or shrimp.

Tips:
The zucchini noodles can get mushy if they are overcooked, so take care not to do that. Simmer them just long enough to be soft, but not so long that they get crispy.

You can customize the pesto sauce by adding ingredients like spinach, arugula, kale, sun-dried tomatoes, or lemon zest for additional flavor and nutrition.

For a dairy-free or vegan version of the pesto sauce, simply omit the Parmesan cheese or replace it with nutritional yeast for a cheesy flavor.

Leftover zucchini noodles with pesto can be stored in an airtight container in the refrigerator for up to 2-3 days. Reheat gently in the microwave or enjoy the cold as a refreshing salad.

Pesto-crusted zucchini noodles are a tasty and adaptable recipe that's ideal for a light lunch or dinner. These colorful, flavorful, and nutrient-dense veggies will quickly become a go-to in your arsenal of healthy vegetable recipes.

Stuffed Bell Peppers with Quinoa and Black Beans

Stuffed bell peppers with quinoa and black beans are a nutritious and satisfying dish that combines the sweetness of bell peppers with the hearty texture of quinoa and the protein-rich goodness of black beans. Here's how to make them:

Ingredients:

Cut four large bell peppers (any color) in half and remove the seeds.
One cup of washed quinoa
One can (15 oz) of rinsed and drained black beans
1 cup corn kernels (fresh, frozen, or canned)
1 small onion, diced
2 cloves garlic, minced
1 teaspoon ground cumin
1 teaspoon chili powder
1/2 teaspoon paprika

Salt and black pepper to taste
1 cup shredded cheese (cheddar, Monterey
Jack, or your favorite melting cheese)
Optional toppings: Fresh chopped cilantro,
avocado slices, salsa, sour cream, or Greek
yogurt.

Instructions:

Preheat Oven: Preheat your oven to 375°F
(190°C). Arrange the halved bell peppers in a
large baking dish, cut side up.

To cook quinoa, place two cups of water in a
medium pot and bring to a boil. Turn down the
heat and add the rinsed quinoa. For fifteen to
twenty minutes, or until the quinoa is cooked
and the water has been absorbed, cover and
simmer. Take off the heat and use a fork to
fluff.

Prepare Filling: In a large skillet, heat olive oil over medium heat. Add diced onion and minced garlic, and sauté until softened, about 3-4 minutes. Add ground cumin, chili powder, paprika, salt, and black pepper, and stir to combine. Add black beans and corn kernels, and cook for an additional 2-3 minutes.

Mix Quinoa and Filling: Combine the black bean and corn mixture in a skillet with the cooked quinoa. To enable the flavors to merge together, simmer, stirring well, for a further two to three minutes. If necessary, taste and adjust the seasoning.

Stuff Bell Peppers: Spoon the quinoa and black bean filling into the halved bell peppers, pressing down gently to pack the filling into each pepper. Fill each pepper generously, dividing the filling evenly among them.

Bake: Evenly cover each stuffed bell pepper with shredded cheese by scattering it on top. When the oven is ready, bake the baking dish covered with aluminum foil for 25 to 30 minutes, or until the cheese is melted and bubbling and the peppers are soft.

To serve, take the filled bell peppers out of the oven and allow them to cool a little. If preferred, garnish with avocado slices, salsa, sour cream, or Greek yogurt along with freshly cut cilantro.

Tips:
You can customize the filling by adding other ingredients such as diced tomatoes, spinach, mushrooms, or cooked ground meat (like turkey or chicken).

For a vegan version, omit the cheese or use a plant-based cheese alternative.

Leftover stuffed bell peppers can be stored in an airtight container in the refrigerator for up to 3-4 days.

Before serving, gently reheat them in the oven or microwave.

Stuffed bell peppers with quinoa and black beans are a flavorful and wholesome meal that's perfect for a satisfying dinner. With their vibrant colors, robust flavors, and nutritious ingredients, they're sure to be a hit with your family and friends.

Eggplant Parmesan

Eggplant Parmesan is a classic Italian dish that features thinly sliced eggplant, breaded and fried until golden, layered with marinara sauce, and baked until bubbly and delicious. Here's how to make a healthier version of this comforting dish:

Ingredients:
2 large eggplants, sliced into 1/2-inch rounds
2 eggs, beaten (or substitute with egg replacer for a vegan version)
1 cup whole wheat breadcrumbs (or gluten-free breadcrumbs)
1/2 cup grated Parmesan cheese (or nutritional yeast for a vegan version)
2 cups marinara sauce (homemade or store-bought)
1 cup shredded mozzarella cheese (or dairy-free mozzarella for a vegan version)
Salt and black pepper to taste
Fresh basil leaves for garnish (optional).

Instructions:

Oven Prep: Set the oven's temperature to 400°F, or 200°C. Apply cooking spray or olive oil sparingly to a baking sheet.

Slices of eggplant should be prepared by placing them on a baking sheet covered with paper towels. To relieve excess moisture, sprinkle salt on both sides and allow to sit for approximately fifteen minutes. Using paper towels, pat the slices of eggplant dry.

Bread Eggplant Slices: In a shallow dish, combine the whole wheat breadcrumbs with the grated Parmesan cheese. Dip each eggplant slice into the beaten eggs (or egg replacer) and then dredge it in the breadcrumb mixture, coating both sides evenly.

Bake Eggplant: Place the breaded eggplant slices on the prepared baking sheet in a single layer. Bake in the preheated oven for 20-25 minutes, flipping halfway through, or until the eggplant slices are golden and crispy.

Assemble Eggplant Parmesan: Spread a thin layer of marinara sauce on the bottom of a baking dish. Arrange half of the baked eggplant slices in a single layer on top of the sauce. Top with more marinara sauce and sprinkle with shredded mozzarella cheese. Repeat with the remaining eggplant slices, marinara sauce, and mozzarella cheese.

Bake: Bake the baking dish in the preheated oven for 25 to 30 minutes, or until the cheese is bubbling and melted, covered with aluminum foil.

Serve: Remove the foil from the baking dish and garnish the eggplant Parmesan with fresh basil leaves, if desired. Serve hot as a main course, accompanied by a side of whole wheat pasta or a green salad.

Tips:
To make this dish even healthier, you can skip the breading and frying step for the eggplant slices. Simply brush the eggplant rounds with olive oil and roast them in the oven until tender.

Use homemade marinara sauce or look for store-bought marinara sauce with no added sugar or preservatives.

For a vegan version, use plant-based ingredients such as nutritional yeast, vegan mozzarella cheese, and egg replacer.

Remaining eggplant For a maximum of three to four days, parmesan can be kept in the refrigerator in an airtight container. Before serving, reheat it in the microwave or oven.

A tasty and filling dish like eggplant parmesan is ideal for a cozy evening at home. Both vegans and meat lovers will love it for its crispy eggplant pieces, rich marinara sauce, and oozy melted cheese.

Lentil and Vegetable Curry

Lentil and vegetable curry is a hearty and nutritious dish that combines protein-rich lentils with an assortment of vegetables in a flavorful and aromatic curry sauce. Here's how to make it:

Ingredients:
One cup of washed and drained dried lentils, either brown or green
2 tablespoons olive oil or coconut oil
1 onion, diced
2 cloves garlic, minced
1 tablespoon fresh ginger, grated
2 carrots, diced
2 potatoes, diced
1 bell pepper, diced
1 cup cauliflower florets
1 cup green peas (fresh or frozen)

2 tablespoons curry powder
1 teaspoon ground cumin
1 teaspoon ground coriander
1/2 teaspoon turmeric powder
1/4 teaspoon cayenne pepper (optional, for heat)
1 can (14 oz) coconut milk
1 can (14 oz) diced tomatoes
Salt and black pepper to taste
Fresh cilantro leaves for garnish (optional)
Cooked rice or naan bread for serving.

Instructions:

Cook Lentils: Rinse the lentils and add enough water to cover them by approximately 2 inches into a big pot. When the water reaches a boil, lower the heat to medium-low and simmer the lentils, uncovered, for 20 to 25 minutes, or until they are soft but not falling apart. After removing any extra water, set away.

To prepare the vegetables, heat the olive oil in a large skillet or pot over medium heat. Cook for approximately five minutes, or until the diced onion is tender. Cook for a further one to two minutes, or until fragrant, after adding the grated ginger and minced garlic.

Add Vegetables and Spices: To the skillet with the sautéed onion, garlic, and ginger, add the chopped carrots, potatoes, bell pepper, cauliflower florets, and green peas. Add the cayenne pepper (if using), turmeric powder, ground cumin, ground coriander, and curry powder and stir. Cook, stirring occasionally, until the veggies start to soften, about 5 to 7 minutes.

Add the diced tomatoes and their juices, along with the coconut milk, and simmer the curry. Mix thoroughly to blend. After bringing the mixture to a simmer, lower the heat to a low setting and cover the pan.

Simmer the curry for fifteen to twenty minutes, or until the flavors have combined and the vegetables are soft.

Combine Lentils and Curry: Put the cooked lentils and the veggie curry in a skillet. Gently mix to blend and fully warm. To taste, add salt and black pepper for seasoning.

Serve: If wanted, top the hot lentil and vegetable curry with fresh cilantro leaves. Serve with naan bread on the side or over cooked rice.

Tips:
Feel free to alter the vegetables to suit your tastes and what you have available. Additional veggies that are excellent in this curry are squash, zucchini, eggplant, kale, and spinach.

Adjust the amount of curry powder and cayenne pepper to suit your desired level of spiciness.

You may keep leftover lentil and vegetable curry in the fridge for up to three to four days if you put it in an airtight container. Before serving, gently reheat in the microwave or on the stove.

Curry made with lentils and vegetables is a tasty and filling recipe that's ideal for a casual dinner any night of the week. Full of fiber, protein, and other nutrients from the lentils and veggies, it's a wholesome and nutrient-dense option that will definitely satisfy your palate.

CHAPTER EIGHT

Baked Vegetable Delight

Baked vegetable delight is a nutritious and flavorful dish that combines a variety of vegetables with herbs, spices, and sometimes cheese, baked until tender and golden. Here's a basic recipe for baked vegetable delight:

Ingredients:
Assorted vegetables (such as bell peppers, zucchini, yellow squash, eggplant, carrots, broccoli, cauliflower, cherry tomatoes, etc.), washed and chopped into bite-sized pieces
Olive oil or avocado oil
Salt and black pepper to taste
Garlic powder, onion powder, dried herbs (such as thyme, rosemary, oregano, or basil), and/or spices (such as paprika, cumin, or chili

powder) to taste
Grated Parmesan cheese or nutritional yeast
(optional).

Instructions:
Preheat Oven: Preheat your oven to 400°F
(200°C). Lightly grease a baking sheet or
roasting pan with olive oil or line it with
parchment paper for easy cleanup.

Prepare Vegetables: Wash and chop the
assorted vegetables into bite-sized pieces. You
can use any combination of vegetables you
like, depending on your preferences and what
you have on hand.

Season Vegetables: In a large mixing bowl,
toss the chopped vegetables with olive oil until
evenly coated. Season with salt, black pepper,
garlic powder, onion powder, dried herbs,
and/or spices according to your taste
preferences. Toss well to coat the vegetables
evenly with the seasoning.

Arrange on Baking Sheet: Spread the seasoned vegetables in a single layer on the prepared baking sheet or roasting pan. Make sure the vegetables are not overcrowded to ensure even cooking and browning.

Bake: Transfer the baking sheet to the preheated oven and bake the vegetables for 20-25 minutes, or until they are tender and golden brown, stirring halfway through cooking to ensure even browning.

Optional Cheese Topping: In the final five minutes of cooking, top the baked vegetables with grated Parmesan cheese or nutritional yeast, if preferred. Place the baking sheet back in the oven and continue baking for another two to three minutes, or until the cheese is bubbling and melted.

To serve, take the cooked veggies out of the oven and allow them to cool a little. Serve hot as an appetizer or side dish to your preferred entrée.

Tips:
Feel free to customize the seasoning and spices according to your taste preferences. You can experiment with different herb and spice combinations to create unique flavor profiles.

Make sure to cut the vegetables into uniform-sized pieces to ensure even cooking.

For a vegan version, omit the cheese topping or use a dairy-free cheese alternative.

Leftover baked vegetables can be stored in an airtight container in the refrigerator for up to 3-4 days. Reheat them gently in the oven or microwave before serving.

Spinach and Feta Stuffed Portobello Mushrooms

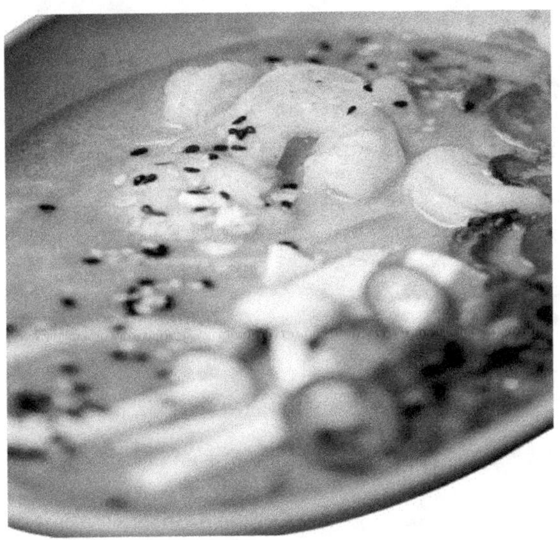

Spinach and feta stuffed portobello mushrooms are a delicious and nutritious dish that features large portobello mushroom caps filled with a savory mixture of spinach, feta cheese, onions, garlic, and herbs. Here's how to make them:

Ingredients:

Four large portobello mushrooms with the gills scraped out and the stems removed

Two tsp olive oil

two minced garlic cloves

One little onion, diced finely

4 cups chopped fresh spinach leaves and 1/2 cup of feta cheese crumbles

To taste, add salt and black pepper.

Not required: For spice, add red pepper flakes.

For garnish, use fresh parsley or basil leaves.

Instructions:

Oven Prep: Set the oven's temperature to 375°F, or 190°C. For easier cleanup, line a baking pan with aluminum foil or parchment paper.

Prepare Mushrooms: Remove the stems from the portobello mushrooms and use a spoon to scrape out the gills from the underside of the caps. Place the cleaned mushroom caps on the prepared baking sheet, gill side up.

Prepare Filling: In a large skillet, heat the olive oil over medium heat. Add the minced garlic and chopped onion, and sauté until softened and fragrant, about 3-4 minutes.

Add Spinach: Add the chopped spinach to the skillet and cook, stirring occasionally, until wilted and tender, about 2-3 minutes.

Season and Combine: Season the spinach mixture with salt, black pepper, and optional red pepper flakes for heat. Stir in the crumbled feta cheese and cook for an additional 1-2 minutes, until the cheese is melted and well incorporated into the mixture.

Stuff Mushrooms: Spoon the spinach and feta mixture into the mushroom caps, dividing it evenly among them and pressing down gently to pack the filling.

Bake: Transfer the stuffed portobello mushrooms to the preheated oven and bake for 20-25 minutes, or until the mushrooms are tender and the filling is heated through.

To serve, take the stuffed portobello mushrooms out of the oven and allow them to cool a little. If desired, garnish with fresh parsley or basil leaves.

Tips:
Choose large, firm portobello mushrooms with smooth caps for the best results.

You can customize the filling by adding other ingredients such as sun-dried tomatoes, chopped olives, or roasted red peppers for additional flavor and texture.

For a dairy-free or vegan version, you can substitute the feta cheese with a dairy-free cheese alternative or omit it altogether.

Leftover stuffed portobello mushrooms can be stored in an airtight container in the refrigerator for up to 2-3 days. Reheat them gently in the oven or microwave before serving.

Stuffed portobello mushrooms with spinach and feta are a tasty and filling dish that's ideal for a light lunch or dinner. They will delight both meat eaters and vegans with their flavorful feta cheese, bright spinach, and earthy mushrooms.

Baked Zucchini Fries

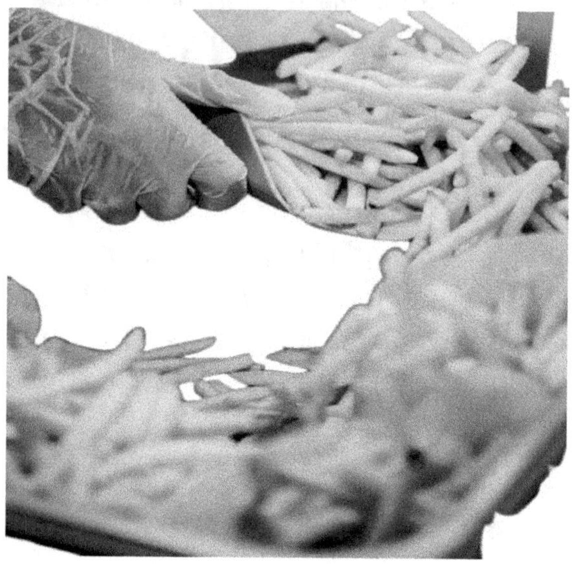

Compared to classic deep-fried french fries, baked zucchini fries are a healthier option because they have a crispy outside and a tender interior because of the zucchini's inherent sweetness. This is how to prepare them:

Ingredients:

Components: two medium zucchini
Half a cup of whole wheat (or gluten-free)
breadcrumbs
1/4 cup of optionally grated Parmesan cheese
one tsp powdered garlic
One dry herbs (such thyme, basil, or oregano)
Half a teaspoon of paprika
To taste, add salt and black pepper.
Two beaten eggs (for a vegan variation, use an
egg replacer)
Cooking spray or olive oil.

Instructions:
Oven Prep: Set the oven's temperature to
425°F (220°C). For easier cleanup, line a
baking pan with aluminum foil or parchment
paper.

Prepare Zucchini: Wash the zucchini and cut
off the ends. Slice the zucchini lengthwise into
thin strips, resembling french fries.

Prepare Coating Mixture: In a shallow dish,
combine the whole wheat breadcrumbs with

grated Parmesan cheese (if using), garlic powder, dried herbs, paprika, salt, and black pepper. Mix well to combine.

Coat Zucchini Strips: Dip each zucchini strip into the beaten eggs (or egg replacer) and then dredge it in the breadcrumb mixture, coating it evenly on all sides. Press gently to adhere the breadcrumbs to the zucchini.

Arrange on Baking Sheet: Place the coated zucchini strips in a single layer on the prepared baking sheet, leaving space between each strip to allow for even cooking.

Bake: Drizzle or spray the zucchini strips lightly with olive oil or cooking spray to help them crisp up in the oven. Bake in the preheated oven for 20-25 minutes, or until the zucchini fries are golden brown and crispy, flipping halfway through cooking for even browning.

Serve: Remove the baked zucchini fries from the oven and let them cool slightly before serving. Serve hot as a healthy and delicious snack or side dish.

Tips:
For extra flavor, you can add additional seasonings to the breadcrumb mixture, such as onion powder, smoked paprika, or Italian seasoning.

Make sure to slice the zucchini into uniform-sized strips to ensure even cooking. For a vegan version, omit the Parmesan cheese or use a dairy-free cheese alternative.

Leftover baked zucchini fries can be stored in an airtight container in the refrigerator for up to 2-3 days. Reheat them in the oven or toaster oven to crisp them up before serving.

Baked zucchini fries are a tasty and nutritious alternative to traditional french fries, offering a satisfying crunch and plenty of flavor without the excess oil and calories. They're perfect for enjoying as a snack, appetizer, or side dish, and they're sure to be a hit with both kids and adults alike.

Stuffed Acorn Squash with Wild Rice

Stuffed acorn squash with wild rice is a delightful and nutritious dish that combines the natural sweetness of acorn squash with hearty wild rice and a variety of flavorful ingredients. Here's how to create this delicious meal:

Ingredients:
2 acorn squash, halved and seeds removed
1 cup wild rice, rinsed
2 cups vegetable broth or water
1 tablespoon olive oil
1 small onion, diced
2 cloves garlic, minced
2 celery stalks, diced
1 carrot, diced
1/2 cup dried cranberries or chopped dried apricots

1/4 cup chopped pecans or walnuts (optional)
2 tablespoons chopped fresh parsley or thyme
Salt and black pepper to taste
Optional toppings: Crumbled feta cheese, goat cheese, or toasted pumpkin seeds.

Instructions:

Oven Prep: Set the oven's temperature to 375°F, or 190°C. For easier cleanup, line a baking pan with aluminum foil or parchment paper.

To prepare the acorn squash, cut it in half lengthwise and use a spoon to remove the stringy pulp and seeds. Squash halves should be placed on the prepared baking sheet, cut side down. Bake for 25 to 30 minutes in a preheated oven, or until a fork inserted into the squash comes out soft.

Cook the wild rice by rinsing it and adding water or vegetable broth to a medium pot. After bringing the liquid to a boil, lower the heat to a simmer, cover the pot, and let the rice cook for 40 to 45 minutes, or until it is soft and the liquid has been completely absorbed. Take off the heat source and use a fork to fluff the rice.

To prepare the filling, heat the olive oil in a large skillet over medium heat. Add the carrot, celery, minced garlic, and diced onion. Sauté the veggies for five to seven minutes, or until they become tender.

Combine Ingredients: Combine the sautéed vegetables and cooked wild rice in a skillet. Add the chopped pecans or walnuts (if using), chopped fresh parsley or thyme, and dried cranberries or chopped dried apricots. To taste, add salt and black pepper for seasoning. Mix thoroughly to blend.

To stuff the acorn squash, turn the roasted halves over so that the sliced side is facing up. Using a spoon, gently put the wild rice stuffing mixture into each squash half.

Bake Again: Put the stuffed acorn squash halves back in the oven and continue to bake for a further 15 to 20 minutes, or until the squash is gently browned around the edges and the filling is heated through.

Serve: Remove the stuffed acorn squash from the oven and let them cool slightly before serving. Garnish with crumbled feta cheese, goat cheese, or toasted pumpkin seeds, if desired.

Tips:
You can customize the filling by adding other ingredients such as chopped apples, diced bell peppers, or cooked chickpeas for additional flavor and texture.

Before taking the acorn squash out of the oven, make sure to check their doneness. When a fork is inserted into the flesh, it should be soft.

For up to two or three days, leftover stuffed acorn squash can be kept in the refrigerator in an airtight container. Before serving, gently reheat them in the oven or microwave.

A filling and substantial dish ideal for a cozy autumn or winter dinner is stuffed acorn squash with wild rice. It will definitely be a success with your family and friends thanks to the combination of sweet squash, nutty wild rice, and savory contents. Savor this filling and tasty dish for any occasion, either as a main course or a side!

Veggie Shepherd's Pie

Veggie Shepherd's Pie is a hearty and wholesome dish that's a vegetarian twist on the classic Shepherd's Pie. Instead of using meat, this recipe features a flavorful mixture of vegetables, lentils, and savory gravy, topped with creamy mashed potatoes and baked until golden and bubbly. Here's how to make it:

Ingredients:

For the Filling:
1 cup of washed and drained lentils, either brown or green
2 cups vegetable broth or water
2 tablespoons olive oil
1 onion, diced
2 cloves garlic, minced
2 carrots, diced
2 celery stalks, diced
1 cup mushrooms, chopped

1 cup frozen peas
1 teaspoon dried thyme
1 teaspoon dried rosemary
Salt and black pepper to taste
2 tablespoons tomato paste
2 tablespoons all-purpose flour or cornstarch
(for thickening)
1 cup vegetable broth or water
For the Mashed Potato Topping:
4 large potatoes, peeled and chopped
1/4 cup unsweetened almond milk or vegetable
broth
2 tablespoons vegan butter or olive oil
Salt and black pepper to taste.

Instructions:
Cook Lentils: In a medium saucepan, combine
the rinsed lentils with 2 cups of vegetable broth
or water. Bring to a boil, then reduce the heat
to low, cover, and simmer for 20-25 minutes, or
until the lentils are tender and the liquid is
absorbed.

Prepare Mashed Potatoes: Put the chopped potatoes in a big pot of water and simmer while the lentils are cooking. After bringing to a boil, lower the heat to medium and simmer the potatoes for 15 to 20 minutes, or until they are tender to the fork. After draining, add the potatoes to a mixing dish. To make the potatoes smooth and creamy, mash them with almond milk, vegetable broth, vegan butter, olive oil, salt, and black pepper. Put aside.

To prepare the filling, place a large skillet over medium heat with olive oil. Cook for approximately five minutes, or until the diced onion is tender. Cook the diced carrots, diced celery, and minced garlic for a further five minutes, or until the veggies are soft. Add the frozen peas, salt, black pepper, dried thyme, and dried rosemary. Chop the mushrooms. Cook for another five minutes, stirring now and then.

Thicken the Gravy: Stir in the tomato paste until well combined. Sprinkle the flour or cornstarch over the vegetable mixture and stir to coat. Cook for 1-2 minutes, then gradually pour in 1 cup of vegetable broth or water, stirring constantly. Cook for another 2-3 minutes, or until the gravy has thickened.

Combine Lentils and Vegetable Mixture: Add the cooked lentils to the skillet with the vegetable mixture. Stir well to combine, then remove from heat.

Put the Shepherd's Pie together: Turn the oven on to 375°F, or 190°C. Spread the lentil and vegetable mixture equally in a large baking dish after transferring it there. Using a spatula to cover the entire surface, spoon the mashed potatoes over the top of the contents.

Bake: Place the baking dish in the preheated oven and bake for 25-30 minutes, or until the mashed potatoes are golden brown and the filling is bubbling around the edges.

Serve: Remove the Veggie Shepherd's Pie from the oven and let it cool for a few minutes before serving. Serve hot, garnished with fresh chopped parsley or thyme, if desired.

Tips:
Feel free to add your preferred veggies or herbs to the stuffing. To add more texture and protein, you can also add cooked beans or lentils.

To make the gravy thicker without gluten, use cornstarch rather than all-purpose flour.

You may keep leftover veggie shepherd's pie in the fridge for up to three or four days if you store it in an airtight container. Before serving, reheat each portion in the oven or microwave.

A filling and healthy recipe, veggie shepherd's pie is ideal for big occasions or cozy weeknight dinners. It's going to become a family favorite with its creamy mashed potato topping and rich, delicious filling!

CHAPTER NINE

Sweet Treats with Vegetables

Sweet treats with vegetables are a creative way to incorporate more nutrition into your desserts while still satisfying your sweet tooth. By using vegetables like carrots, zucchini, sweet potatoes, pumpkin, or beets, you can add moisture, sweetness, and nutrients to your treats.

Carrot Cake: Carrot cake is a classic dessert that uses grated carrots in the batter to add moisture and sweetness. It's typically spiced with cinnamon, nutmeg, and cloves, and often includes nuts and raisins for extra texture. Top it with a creamy cream cheese frosting for the perfect finish.

Zucchini Bread: Zucchini bread is a moist and flavorful quick bread made with grated zucchini. The zucchini adds moisture and tenderness to the bread, while spices like cinnamon and nutmeg give it warmth and flavor. It's perfect for breakfast, snack time, or dessert.

Sweet Potato Brownies: Sweet potato brownies are a healthier alternative to traditional brownies, with mashed sweet potatoes adding moisture and natural sweetness. They're fudgy, chocolatey, and delicious, making them a guilt-free treat.

Pumpkin Muffins: Pumpkin muffins are moist and tender muffins made with pureed pumpkin. They're flavored with warm spices like cinnamon, ginger, and cloves, and are perfect for enjoying during the fall months or any time of year.

Beet Chocolate Cake: Beet chocolate cake is a rich and decadent chocolate cake made with pureed beets. The beets add moisture and a subtle earthy sweetness to the cake, while cocoa powder provides rich chocolate flavor. It's a delicious way to sneak some veggies into your dessert.

Avocado Chocolate Mousse: Avocado chocolate mousse is a creamy and indulgent dessert made with ripe avocados, cocoa powder, and sweetener. The avocado gives the mousse its silky texture and adds healthy fats, while the cocoa powder provides rich chocolate flavor. It's a decadent treat that's also packed with nutrients.

Spinach Smoothie Popsicles: Blend spinach leaves with fruits like banana, pineapple, and mango, along with some yogurt or coconut milk, then pour the mixture into popsicle molds and freeze for a healthy and refreshing treat.

Carrot Cake Muffins

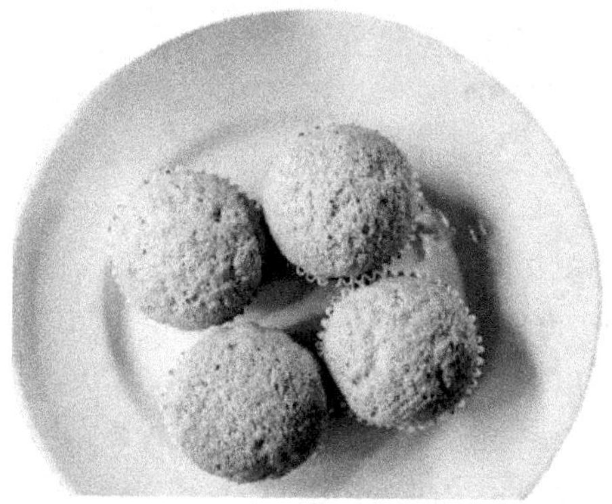

Carrot cake muffins are a delightful twist on the classic carrot cake, offering all the flavors of the beloved dessert in portable, individual servings. These muffins are moist, tender, and bursting with the natural sweetness of carrots, making them a perfect treat for breakfast, snack time, or dessert. Here's how to make these healthy and delicious carrot cake muffins:

Ingredients:
1 1/2 cups of whole wheat flour (or a blend of
flour without gluten)
1 teaspoon baking powder
1/2 teaspoon baking soda
1/2 teaspoon ground cinnamon
1/4 teaspoon ground nutmeg
1/4 teaspoon ground ginger
1/4 teaspoon salt
1/4 cup coconut oil or melted butter
1/2 cup maple syrup or honey
2 large eggs
1 teaspoon vanilla extract
1 1/2 cups grated carrots (about 2-3 medium
carrots)
1/2 cup chopped walnuts or pecans (optional)
1/4 cup raisins or chopped dried apricots
(optional).

Instructions:
Oven Prep: Set the oven's temperature to
350°F, or 175°C. Use cooking spray or paper
liners to line a muffin tray.

Prepare Dry Ingredients: In a large mixing bowl, whisk together the whole wheat flour, baking powder, baking soda, cinnamon, nutmeg, ginger, and salt until well combined. Set aside.

Mix Wet Ingredients: In another bowl, whisk together the melted coconut oil or butter, maple syrup or honey, eggs, and vanilla extract until smooth and well combined.

Mix Wet and Dry components: Add the wet components to the dry ones in a bowl, stirring to mix them together just enough. Take caution not to blend too much. When the carrots are grated and the nuts, if any, are chopped, fold them into the dough until the raisins or dried apricots are uniformly distributed.

Fill Muffin Cups: Evenly distribute the batter into the muffin cups that have been prepared, filling each to about two-thirds of the way.

Bake: For 18 to 20 minutes, or until the muffins are golden brown and a toothpick inserted into the center comes out clean, place the muffin tin in the preheated oven.

Cool and Serve: Remove the muffins from the oven and let them cool in the pan for a few minutes before transferring them to a wire rack to cool completely. Serve the carrot cake muffins warm or at room temperature.

Tips:
For a gluten-free version, use a gluten-free flour blend in place of whole wheat flour.

Feel free to customize the muffins by adding your favorite mix-ins such as shredded coconut, chopped pineapple, or crushed pineapple.

Leftover muffins can be frozen for longer storage or kept at room temperature for up to three days in an airtight container. Before serving, reheat the thawed muffins in the oven or microwave.

These carrot cake muffins are the ideal snack for any time of day since they are tasty, moist, and full of healthy ingredients. Savor them as a filling snack, a healthy breakfast on the run, or a guilt-free dessert.

Zucchini Bread

Zucchini bread is a moist and flavorful quick bread that incorporates grated zucchini into the batter, adding both moisture and natural sweetness. This recipe is a great way to use up surplus zucchini from the garden and sneak some extra veggies into your diet. Here's how to make zucchini bread:

Ingredients:
About two medium zucchini, or two cups of shredded zucchini
One and a half cups all-purpose flour (for a healthy choice, use whole wheat flour)
Half a cup of granulated sugar (for a refined sugar-free alternative, use coconut sugar, honey, or maple syrup)
Half a cup of dense brown sugar
Melted coconut oil or half a cup of vegetable oil
2 large eggs
1 teaspoon vanilla extract
1 teaspoon ground cinnamon

1/2 teaspoon ground nutmeg
1/2 teaspoon baking soda
1/2 teaspoon baking powder
1/2 teaspoon salt
Optional mix-ins: chopped nuts, raisins, dried cranberries, or chocolate chips.

Instructions:

Oven Prep: Set the oven's temperature to 350°F, or 175°C. For easier removal, line a 9x5-inch loaf pan with parchment paper or grease it.

Prepare the zucchini by grating it with a food processor or box grater. After grating the zucchini, place it in a fresh kitchen towel and press off any extra moisture. Put aside.

Mix Wet Ingredients: In a large mixing bowl, whisk together the granulated sugar, brown sugar, vegetable oil, eggs, and vanilla extract until well combined and smooth.

Combine Dry Ingredients: In a separate bowl, whisk together the flour, cinnamon, nutmeg, baking soda, baking powder, and salt until well combined.

Mix Wet and Dry Ingredients: Stir the dry ingredients into the wet ones only until they are well blended. Add the dry ingredients gradually. Once the grated zucchini and any optional mix-ins (such chocolate chips or almonds) are thoroughly mixed into the batter, fold them in.

Bake: Evenly spread out the batter after pouring it into the loaf pan. Bake for 50–60 minutes in a preheated oven, or until the top is golden brown and a toothpick inserted in the center comes out clean.

Cool: After taking the zucchini bread out of the oven, leave it in the pan for ten to fifteen minutes. Before slicing, carefully move it to a wire rack to cool entirely.

Serve: Slice the zucchini bread and serve it warm or at room temperature. Enjoy it plain, with a smear of butter or cream cheese, or toasted for extra flavor.

Tips:
Be sure to properly drain the grated zucchini to remove excess moisture, as this will prevent the bread from becoming soggy.

Feel free to customize the bread by adding your favorite mix-ins, such as chopped nuts, raisins, dried cranberries, or chocolate chips.

Leftover zucchini bread can be frozen for longer storage or kept at room temperature for up to three days in an airtight container. Before serving, thaw frozen slices in the fridge or at room temperature.

Delicious and adaptable, zucchini bread is great for breakfast, as a snack, or as dessert. It is sure to please the whole family with its moist texture and delicate taste!

Sweet Potato Brownies

Sweet potato brownies are a healthier twist on traditional brownies, incorporating the natural sweetness and moisture of sweet potatoes while reducing the amount of refined flour and sugar typically found in classic recipes. These brownies are fudgy, decadent, and packed with nutrients, making them a guilt-free indulgence. Here's how to make them:

Ingredients:
1 cup mashed sweet potatoes (about 2 medium sweet potatoes, cooked and mashed)
1/2 cup almond flour or oat flour
1/4 cup cocoa powder
1/4 cup maple syrup or honey
1/4 cup of unsweetened applesauce or melted coconut oil
Two eggs (vegan option: flax eggs)
One tsp vanilla essence
One-half tsp baking powder
A dash of salt

Chocolate chips, dried fruit, chopped almonds, or shredded coconut are examples of optional mix-ins.

Instructions:
Preheat Oven: Preheat your oven to 350°F (175°C). Grease a 9x9-inch baking pan or line it with parchment paper for easy removal.

Prepare Sweet Potatoes: Wash the sweet potatoes and pierce them several times with a fork. Place them on a baking sheet and bake in the preheated oven for 45-60 minutes, or until they are soft and tender. Let them cool slightly, then peel off the skins and mash the flesh with a fork or potato masher until smooth. Measure out 1 cup of mashed sweet potatoes for the recipe.

Mix Wet Ingredients: In a large mixing bowl, whisk together the mashed sweet potatoes, maple syrup or honey, melted coconut oil or applesauce, eggs (or flax eggs), and vanilla extract until well combined and smooth.

Combine Dry Ingredients: In a separate bowl, whisk together the almond flour or oat flour, cocoa powder, baking powder, and salt until well combined.

Mix Wet and Dry Ingredients: Stir the dry ingredients into the wet ones only until they are well blended. Add the dry ingredients gradually. Take caution not to blend too much. Add any optional mix-ins, such chocolate chips or chopped nuts, and fold until they are uniformly mixed into the mixture.

Bake: Using a spatula, evenly distribute the mixture into the baking pan that has been prepared. When the brownies are set and a toothpick put into the center comes out mainly clean with a few moist crumbs attached, they are baked for 20 to 25 minutes in a preheated oven.

Cool and Serve: Remove the brownies from the oven and let them cool completely in the pan before slicing into squares. Serve the sweet potato brownies at room temperature and enjoy!

Tips:
Be sure to use cooked and mashed sweet potatoes for this recipe. You can roast or boil the sweet potatoes until tender, then mash them with a fork or potato masher.

Feel free to customize the brownies by adding your favorite mix-ins, such as chopped nuts, chocolate chips, dried fruit, or shredded coconut.

Sweet potato brownies leftovers can be kept at room temperature for up to three days in an airtight container, or they can be kept longer in the refrigerator. Savor them as a healthy after-meal alternative or snack!

Rich, fudgy, and gratifying, these sweet potato brownies have a touch of natural sweetness from the sweet potatoes. They're the ideal dessert choice for anyone searching for a healthier alternative because they're a tasty way to satisfy your chocolate cravings while sneaking in some extra nutrients.

Pumpkin Spice Smoothie

A Pumpkin Spice Smoothie is a delicious and nutritious beverage that captures the flavors of autumn with the warm and comforting spices typically found in pumpkin pie. This smoothie combines pumpkin puree, spices, and other ingredients to create a creamy and satisfying drink that's perfect for breakfast, a snack, or even dessert. Here's how to make it:

Ingredients:
1/2 cup pumpkin puree (canned or homemade)
1 ripe banana, frozen
1/2 cup plain Greek yogurt (or dairy-free yogurt for a vegan option)
1/2 cup almond milk, unsweetened (or any other type of milk)
One tablespoon honey or maple syrup, adjusted to taste

1/2 teaspoon ground cinnamon
1/4 teaspoon ground ginger
1/4 teaspoon ground nutmeg
1/8 teaspoon ground cloves
1/2 teaspoon vanilla extract
Handful of ice cubes.

Instructions:
Blend Ingredients: In a blender, combine the pumpkin puree, frozen banana, Greek yogurt, almond milk, maple syrup or honey, ground cinnamon, ground ginger, ground nutmeg, ground cloves, vanilla extract, and ice cubes.

Blend on high speed until the contents are well incorporated and the smoothie has a creamy, smooth consistency. Add a small amount of extra almond milk at a time until the required consistency is achieved if the consistency is too thick.

Taste and Adjust: Taste the smoothie and adjust the sweetness or spice level as needed. You can add more maple syrup or spices according to your preference.

Serve: Pour the pumpkin spice smoothie into glasses and garnish with a sprinkle of ground cinnamon or a dollop of whipped cream if desired. Serve immediately and enjoy!

Tips:
To make the smoothie thicker, you can add more frozen bananas or a handful of ice cubes.

Customize the smoothie by adding protein powder, chia seeds, flaxseeds, or a handful of spinach for extra nutrition.

You can use canned coconut milk in place of almond milk for a creamier texture.

Greek yogurt can be substituted with coconut yogurt or any other non-dairy yogurt if you'd rather eat dairy-free.

A delicious and healthy way to savor the tastes of fall in a refreshing drink is with this Pumpkin Spice Smoothie. It will quickly become a favorite seasonal delicacy thanks to its warming spices and creamy texture!

CONCLUSION

Inclusion, "Healthy Vegetable Recipes for Beginners" offers a comprehensive guide to incorporating more nutritious and delicious vegetable-based dishes into your diet. From vibrant salads to hearty soups, flavorful stir-fries to satisfying main courses, this book provides easy-to-follow recipes that are perfect for novice cooks and seasoned chefs alike.

With an emphasis on fresh, whole ingredients and simple cooking techniques, each recipe is designed to showcase the natural flavors and health benefits of vegetables. Whether you're looking to improve your overall health, lose weight, or simply explore new culinary horizons, this book has something for everyone.

You'll discover a world of flavors and textures that will excite your taste senses and leave you feeling content and nourished by adding more veggies to your meals. You'll also increase your intake of important vitamins, minerals, and fiber.

Therefore, "Healthy Vegetable Recipes for Beginners" is your go-to resource for producing wholesome and delectable meals that will please your senses and promote your well-being for years to come, regardless of your level of culinary experience.

Thank you for exploring "Healthy Vegetable Recipes for Beginners" with us. We hope this culinary journey has inspired you to embrace the power of vegetables and embark on a path towards improved health and well-being.

By choosing to prioritize vegetables in your diet, you're not only nourishing your body with essential nutrients but also supporting a sustainable and eco-friendly food system. Your commitment to incorporating more vegetables into your meals is a powerful step towards creating a healthier future for yourself and the planet.

We appreciate your commitment to savoring new tastes, experimenting with seasonal foods, and using the straightforward act of cooking to take control of your health. By working together, we may build a community of strong, self-assured cooks who are enthusiastic about providing for both their physical and spiritual needs.

We appreciate you coming along on this path to a better, more confident version of yourself. Cheers to a lifetime of strong health and many more delightful culinary explorations. Happy cooking and cheers to you.